FEARLESS MENOPAUSE

FEARLESS
MENOPAUSE

A BODY-POSITIVE GUIDE TO NAVIGATING MIDLIFE CHANGES

Barb DePree, MD

ROCKRIDGE
PRESS

For general information on our other products and services or to obtain technical support, please contact our Customer Care Department within the United States at (866) 744-2665 or outside the United States at (510) 253-0500.

Rockridge Press publishes its books in a variety of electronic and print formats. Some content that appears in print may not be available in electronic books, and vice versa.

Interior and Cover Designer: Regina Stadnik
Art Producer: Samantha Ulban
Editor: Natasha Yglesias
Production Manager: Martin Worthington
Production Editor: Melissa Edeburn

Stephanie Wunderlich/Offset; Bibadash/Shutterstock, cover. All other illustrations used under license © Bibadash/Shutterstock

Author photo courtesy © Colleen Chrzanowski

ISBN: Print 978-1-64152-730-9 | Ebook 978-1-64152-731-6

R0

CONTENTS

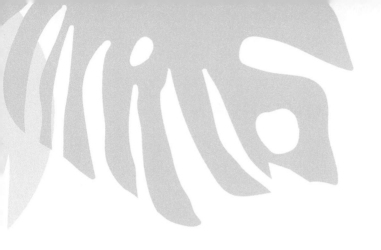

This book is for women everywhere, and especially for my daughters and their generation, in hopes that we'll keep learning to navigate our transitions from positions of knowledge and power.

INTRODUCTION

You've picked up this book because you're noticing changes in yourself or perhaps because of conversations with someone else—a colleague, partner, family member, or friend—about what they're experiencing. Maybe things are changing and you're not sure you understand why. You may be curious about what's happening and what comes next.

As a menopause care provider, I hear questions about these changes every day. Many people are surprised by the signs of approaching menopause. Shockingly few people have had a thorough education on menopause, which means that when menopause arrives, many women have to scramble to decode and treat individual symptoms with no larger picture to provide perspective. Some women feel uncomfortable talking about their symptoms with others, which can lead to discouragement or isolation. To make matters worse, health care providers aren't universally trained to consider the effects of perimenopause and menopause in their diagnostic process.

I began my career as an OB/GYN more than 30 years ago. For the first few decades, I treated women of all ages, diagnosing health issues, monitoring pregnancies, and delivering babies. It was immensely satisfying, albeit difficult to do well while raising three daughters. Fifteen years ago, I stepped back to reevaluate my focus. I saw that midlife women in my community specifically lacked resources to navigate postreproductive health and happiness in an informed, supported way.

So I went back to school. I pursued certification from the North American Menopause Society (NAMS) to become a menopause care specialist. I redesigned my practice to focus specifically on midlife women. Unsurprisingly (to me especially, as I was in perimenopause myself), the practice took off, confirming the need for special attention in this oft-neglected field of health care.

After a few years in that specialized practice, I began to notice another underserved field—female sexual health at midlife and beyond. Many of my patients had concerns about the role of sexual intimacy at this point in their lives and their ability to enjoy it. I couldn't find many informational resources for them, and the few over-the-counter products I knew would be helpful were difficult to get a hold of.

So I launched a website, MiddlesexMD.com, to provide information and specially chosen products to support midlife women and their sexual health. MiddlesexMD has opened doors for me in so many ways: I've been able to review and make suggestions about pharmaceutical companies' research for menopausal women, meet health care leaders who set the standards for medical care, and interview medical and health sciences researchers, practitioners of traditional and nontraditional therapies, and advocates for women's health care. I've corresponded with hundreds of women about their experiences, helping them understand the bigger picture of their health at this stage, and what resources can help them live the lives they choose. After blogging regularly in response to these discussions, I published the book *Yes You Can: Dr. Barb's Recipe for Lifelong Intimacy*. It was the outreach and education I've done through MiddlesexMD that led to my being named Certified Menopause Practitioner of the Year by NAMS in 2013.

I'm a doctor, a wife, a mother to three daughters, and now a grandmother, too. I see patients regularly, in my own practice as well as at the High Risk Breast Clinic, and I serve as the director of midlife women's health for Holland Hospital. I lead a small team at MiddlesexMD, where we continue to spread the word that satisfying intimacy needn't end when menstruation does. On top of all that, I make time for yoga and cycling to manage my own health, too.

From my years of experience, I can affirm one thing: The best place to start addressing menopause symptoms is to learn about the big picture. What's changing, and what are the effects? What's typical, and what's "normal"? When you have an understanding of what's happening in your body and why, you can minimize surprises, listen to what your body is telling you, and get ahead of symptoms before they disrupt your life. You're as strong and capable at this point in your life as you've ever been, and taking (or keeping) control of your health during this transition can help you ensure that you continue to be.

I hope you'll use this book to help you navigate these changes in ways that work for you. I'll define the stages of transition that are collectively called *menopause*. I'll explain how hormonal changes during menopause affect the body and mind, and I'll provide strategies you can use to keep your health in check through the transition and beyond.

Menopause can be disconcerting, difficult, and scary. But menopause also provides freedom: freedom from the discomfort, inconvenience, and even more serious health issues associated with menstrual cycles and from concerns about contraception. For many of us, the menopause transition comes during a time when we are coming into our own. Some of us are seeing changes in our careers, whether through a promotion, a career change, or retirement. Some of us are seeing our families grow or change; others of us are leaving past relationships behind and entering into new relationships. At this point in our lives, we may feel more comfortable being honest about the people and things that are most important to us. Since it intersects with all of these changes and evolutions, I like to think of menopause as an opportunity for reinvention.

Getting the facts is the first step.

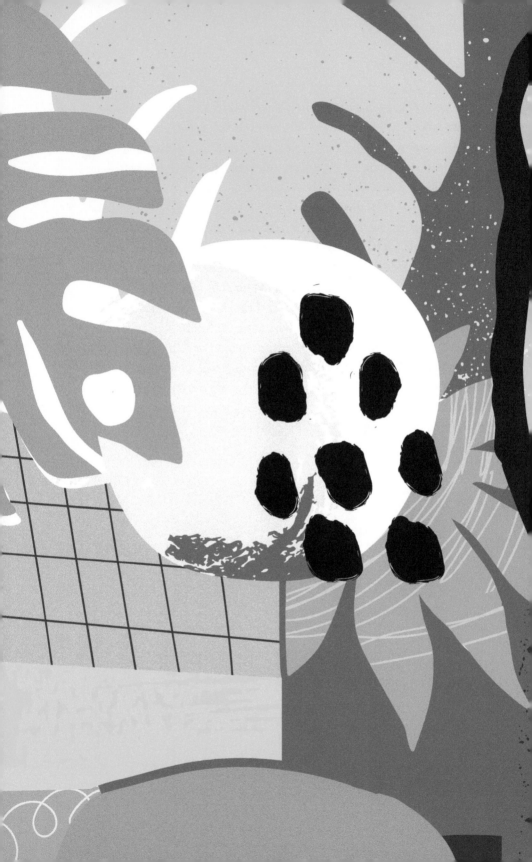

CHAPTER ONE

A NATURAL TIME FOR REINVENTION

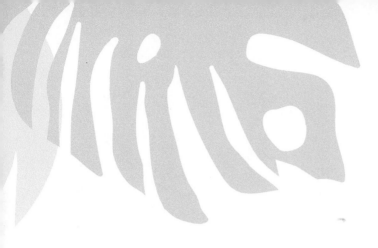

As a woman, a mother of adult daughters, and a menopause care provider, I'm especially aware that what we learn about women's sexual health is almost exclusively limited to puberty and reproduction. Neither I nor my daughters learned anything about menopause in health class, and the questions I get from patients tell me we're not alone.

More informed conversations about menopause will help us change the narrative. Menopause is not a decline—it marks the beginning of another major chapter in our lives, just as empowering and important as the reproductive stage but in different ways. When I talk to patients about the amount of variability they can expect in menopause, I often use pregnancy as an analogy. I can tell them what to expect in a general sense: There is a known process that occurs during pregnancy, labor, and delivery, and at the end, there's a baby. Every journey through that process, though, is different; no one can predict it fully. There could be unanticipated health issues or complications during labor that throw plans for delivery out the window. For some, pregnancy is much easier than expected, and a detailed plan doesn't turn out to be necessary.

When we reach menopause, we know we're moving out of the reproductive years, but the journey will be different for everyone. Some are pleasantly surprised; others, not so much. My goal, both in my practice and in this book, is to help you understand and navigate that journey in ways that work for you.

WHAT IS MENOPAUSE?

The terminology itself is confusing. Menopause is sometimes talked about as though it's a "stage," whereas the reality is that it's a medical milestone and a drawn-out process. The medical milestone is when a woman stops menstruating—that is, once she has no period for a full year. The process is much more protracted (longer lasting) than most are aware. It's not a straight line in any sense—if you mapped hormone levels during menopause, you'd see a jumble. We can't predict the timing. Sometimes you take one step forward and two steps back. Although there is an average age, we don't know exactly when you as an individual can expect to reach menopause.

There are exceptions, of course, like those who have had a "complete" hysterectomy (or hysterectomy with oophorectomy), meaning that ovaries were removed, or those whose ovaries were damaged through another treatment, for example, chemotherapy. Such a procedure can happen at any age and for a variety of medical reasons, and it triggers an abrupt menopause.

WE'RE IN THIS TOGETHER

You're certainly not alone in the menopause transition. About 1.3 million women in the United States alone become menopausal each year. The numbers vary with other demographic indicators, but longer life expectancies mean that more women reach menopause and live for decades thereafter. I've seen the prediction that by 2030, 47 million women around the world will reach this milestone annually. That global study also predicts that Earth's population of postmenopausal women will reach 1.2 billion the same year.

Demographic research is typically based on age (usually 50), which menopause doesn't necessarily respect. The median age for menopause is 51, but the median represents a range of 40 to 60, with a few outside the range. I was recently in a meeting with four women, and the topic of menopause came up. In that group alone, one of us had become menopausal at 39 and another at 60.

THE STAGES

Rather than regarding menopause as one significant event—a year without menstruating—I find it more helpful to break it down into stages between any two of which there's no hard line.

Late Reproductive Years

Although you're still ovulating during your late reproductive years, you're less likely to become pregnant. You may have shorter menstrual cycles, meaning periods may be closer together, and they may be lighter or heavier than usual. In the first week of your cycle, the follicle-stimulating hormone (FSH), which helps your ovary release eggs, may be at a higher level than usual. The rise in FSH is a natural effort on the part of your body to continue to enable reproduction. This stage can last for as long as nine years, but like many other parts of the menopause transition, the duration varies significantly.

Early Menopausal Transition

This stage is the official beginning of perimenopause, when "typical" symptoms of menopause begin: hot flashes, mood swings, interrupted sleep, loss of libido, and vaginal dryness. During this time, the hormones estrogen and progesterone are being produced in fluctuating levels from week to week and even day to day (over time, levels will decline).

During this time, menstrual cycles become more variable, even entirely unpredictable. I like to say that unpredictable is the new normal. PMS symptoms, like bloating and irritability, may increase. Keeping track of your own symptoms during this stage can help your health care provider determine where you are on the transition path.

This stage lasts an average of four years, but of course, it may be shorter or longer.

Late Menopausal Transition

During this stage, the likelihood of typical menopausal symptoms increases, especially hot flashes, interrupted sleep, and mood swings.

During this time, you're likely to miss an entire period or two, and you'll continue to experience the normal unpredictability you've come to know.

If you look at a long-enough line graph, you'll see that hormone production is in decline. Day to day, though, production of estrogen and progesterone can vary wildly. This stage is frequently called the "second half" of perimenopause, but that characterization is not entirely accurate because for most people, it's shorter than the "first half," lasting only a year or two.

Postmenopause

A full year after your last period (the medical milestone), you'll have solidly arrived. Unless you have received hormone therapy, your levels of estrogen and progesterone will be very low by this point. If you haven't experienced them yet, you may have hot flashes, difficulty with sleep, some loss of comfort during or enjoyment of sexual intimacy, or other symptoms. If you've already been dealing with those symptoms, they may get worse for a while.

I often need to explain that there is no "cure" for menopause, just as there is no cure for puberty. Doctors describe it as a chronic condition, meaning it's ongoing and here to stay. Beyond sexual health, menopause affects your bones, your heart, and your brain. That's why I encourage my patients to learn about their bodies and make changes to stay as healthy as they can, physically and emotionally, for the rest of their lives.

Not long ago, life expectancies were shorter, making menopause a rare condition. Many women died before they stopped menstruating, and many more died before experiencing menopause fully. We may be the first generation called on to actively manage our health throughout menopause—but we're lucky to have the opportunity.

A Word about Testing

I know from years of conversations with patients in my practice that they want road maps, definitions, and certainty regarding their health. Many of my patients, wishing to decode their symptoms, ask me whether there's a test that will tell them where they are in this menopause transition.

The answer is yes, there's a blood test that measures FSH level. But I don't recommend it.

The blood test reflects the day you took it, not the entire trend line of hormone production, so the fluctuating hormone levels I mentioned can make the test entirely misleading. You may be 52 with symptoms of perimenopause, but if you happen to take the test the one time in six months that you ovulated, your FSH level will falsely indicate that you're not menopausal.

On top of all that, even before perimenopause, many women have erratic periods and hormone levels. FSH level is also affected by lifestyle factors, like smoking and stress.

Instead of taking that test, I encourage my patients to use a journal to track their own symptoms, from periods to irritability and cramps to insomnia and uncomfortable sex. A few months of journal keeping may be the most helpful tool for you and your doctor to understand where you are in menopause. I'll reference journal keeping as a useful tool throughout this book.

The bottom line is we're humans, not mass-produced machines. Tune in to your body and take the changes a month at a time.

SELF-CARE
BE KIND TO YOURSELF

During this transition, it's valuable to devote extra care to yourself—you need it, but you also deserve it. A healthy diet, regular exercise, and adequate sleep, among other self-care basics, will help as you navigate menopause.

Now is also a time for you to manage stress however is useful for you. Some form of meditation may be helpful. I value my daily yoga, which combines meditation with strength and flexibility training. Try getting outside or spending time in nature. Treat yourself to a spa day. Devote some time to spend with friends or family—community helps us stay grounded during stressful times.

If you don't already, I recommend keeping a journal to keep track of how you're feeling physically and emotionally. A journal provides a tangible reminder to check in with yourself, which is sometimes a new habit for those of us at midlife. Reviewing your journal can help you identify patterns and cause-and-effect relationships. It may help you set boundaries and make it clearer when you need to say no to something (and when you should say yes).

WHAT TO EXPECT

Nearly every woman can expect a series of changes in her menstrual cycle, caused by the retirement of the ovaries' follicle production. During the reproductive years, those follicles produce estrogen that circulates through our bodies, put to use by receptors to serve multiple functions from head to toe. If your periods have always been irregular, if you've had an endometrial ablation (a surgical destruction of the lining of the uterus to manage heavy periods), or if you've had a hysterectomy that left your ovaries in place, you may find it more difficult to judge your progression in the menopausal transition. You may find using a health journal especially valuable to help identify other patterns or signs during this time.

The more difficult prediction to make is *how* your periods will change. They may be further apart or closer together, heavier or lighter, shorter or longer—as I'm sure you've learned by now, it varies. Health factors, age, lifestyle, stress level, and genetics can each shape your individual experience of menopause.

Hot flashes are probably the most common symptom of menopause, but again, there's a lot of variability. For some, a hot flash manifests as a barely noticeable feverish (or sometimes chilly) moment, easily ignored. Others become noticeably flushed, start dripping with sweat, and experience rapid heartbeat. Night sweats are the overnight version of hot flashes, which can sometimes wake you up soaked in sweat.

Without steady levels of estrogen, the urogenital tissues (vulva, vagina, urethra, and lower bladder) begin to regress. The earliest and most common result is vaginal dryness, experienced by 60 percent of women or more. We'll cover this topic in much more detail later.

If you've had emotional symptoms during PMS, you can imagine that the fluctuating hormones of the menopause transition might trigger mood swings. You may have bouts of anger, depression, irritability, or a combination. It can also be difficult to parse what can be attributed to menopause and what's caused by normal stress. Maybe your job is no longer as satisfying as it once was, you need to delay your retirement, or you have to take care of a sick parent. Maybe you're an empty-nester with the blues, a romantic relationship is causing strain, or you're feeling like you missed out on some career or life opportunity. It's always possible that menopause is a factor in whatever you're going through, but don't dismiss your feelings merely as symptoms of menopause. Whatever you're going through, be aware of what you're feeling, address any issues you can, and seek support when you need it.

WHAT IS NORMAL?

I hope it's clear by this point that there's a very broad range of "normal" in the menopause transition. Timing varies, both in age of onset and duration of each stage. You may have lighter or heavier periods more or less frequently. You might have your last period at 39 or 60. You may have hot flashes; they could be severe or hardly noticeable. You may have mood changes or you may not. You could have any number of other symptoms, detailed in the next chapter.

"Normal" is your own definition of your own experience. Doctors don't have a standard set of parameters for when to treat (or not treat) symptoms of perimenopause or menopause. I tell my patients that when a symptom is disruptive to them, we can explore options to address it. Returning to the pregnancy analogy, there are endless ways to reach the goal, but the journey will always vary from person to person. My job as a health care provider is to make the journey as navigable as possible.

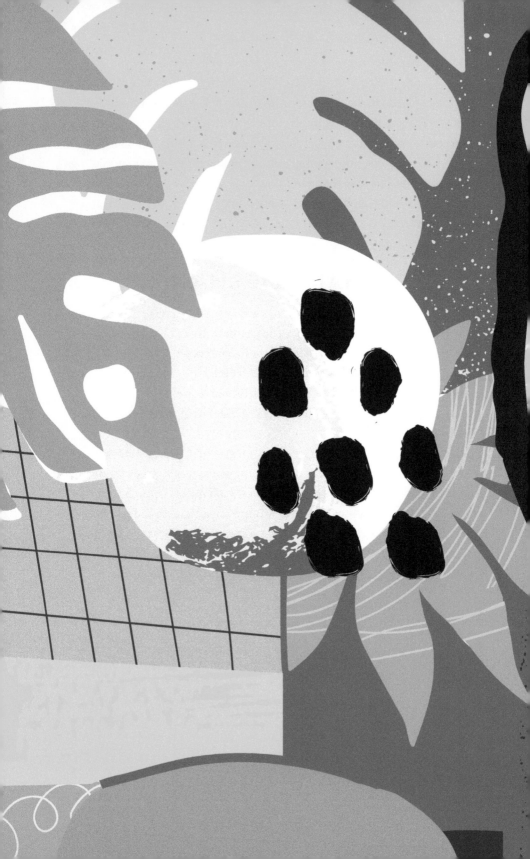

CHAPTER TWO

BODY AND MIND CHANGES DURING "THE CHANGE"

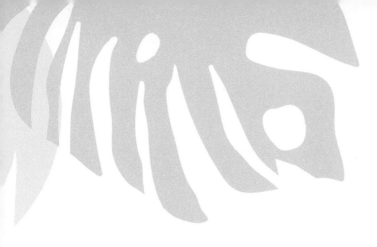

Your body is beautiful and capable of amazing things—that fact hasn't changed, and it won't change now. There are some things that will change, however, which I'll explain through the lens of hormones.

HORMONES RULE

Let's start with a quick science lesson. Think of hormones as "chemical messengers" for your body. Hormones are produced by a number of organs, including the heart, kidneys, pancreas, intestines, and ovaries. Hormones travel from where they're produced to cells in other parts of our bodies, which are activated by the chemical messages the hormones contain. Female bodies actually have 50 or so hormones, but just a handful change with menopause. When puberty begins, FSH levels increase, signaling the ovaries to produce estrogen (and progesterone). During menopause, the level of estrogen drops, typically to about 1 percent of its original level.

Let's start with a primer on estrogen. Estrogen is a small family of hormones that includes estradiol, estriol, and estrone. Estradiol is produced by our ovaries and plays a dominant role during our reproductive years. Estriol is primarily relevant in pregnancy. Estrone is usually produced by fat—or by converted estradiol circulating throughout the body—and dominates postmenopause.

Estrogen effects the entire body throughout life because of proteins inside of cells called *estrogen receptors*. Estrogen receptors are in your brain, bones, heart, skin, genitals, lungs, liver—nearly everywhere. When the estrogen and the receptor combine, they work to manage cell growth and quality or to regulate function.

During puberty, estrogen spurs the development of secondary sex characteristics, like breasts, (widening) hips, and pubic and armpit hair. In combination with other hormones, estrogen helps the fallopian tubes, vagina, and uterus develop. It also manages the menstrual cycle. Estrogen supports bone and skin health, too. It regulates the liver in producing cholesterol, which contributes to heart health. We know it plays an important, though not entirely understood, role in the brain, as well.

Now, let's take a look at FSH and how it interacts with estrogen. During the reproductive years, the pituitary gland sends out FSH to trigger the ovaries to make estrogen and progesterone. Estrogen helps eggs grow and the lining of the uterus thicken. If our estrogen level is low because we're becoming menopausal (and concluding production), the pituitary gland will release more FSH to trigger the ovaries to make more estrogen (and progesterone, which plays a critical role during pregnancy and nursing and is also believed to be the trigger for PMS symptoms, like bloating, tender breasts, and moodiness). This FSH activity can lead to the sudden spikes and drops in hormone levels that are associated with menopause.

If you were to make a line graph of FSH, estrogen, and progesterone levels from postpuberty until the start of perimenopause, the graph would show clear, consistent cycles, with estrogen, progesterone, and FSH each repeating their own pattern of rising and falling levels (unless, of course, you've had irregular periods your whole life). Once you enter perimenopause, the lines are more likely to look like a ball of yarn a kitten has played with: You may not be able to see defined cycles, and the three hormones will likely fluctuate without a clear relationship to one another.

The unpredictability and individuality of the menopause transition can be attributed to the interactions among multiple hormones, each of which has a specific role to play and has its own impact when its level changes.

FIRST SIGNS

As mentioned previously, women usually first notice a change in their menstrual cycle. Other signs of perimenopause often go unnoticed either because they're mild or because they're attributed to something else. A shift in sexual desire, for example, might be chalked up to exhaustion from overcommitment or a busy schedule. You could blame insomnia on money troubles, worrisome colleagues, a heavy workload, or other sources of stress. You may think you're forgetful because you've got too much on your plate to stay on top of it all. And honestly, all of those things could be true. But you could also be perimenopausal.

I'm not sure if it's because of midwestern practicality or physician's pragmatism, but if I could, I'd shift the way we think about the menopause transition. Unless an unusual health event or medical intervention changes our path, we're all headed toward perimenopause and then menopause. There are so many variables in our experiences of each stage, I'm not sure how helpful it is to try to pigeonhole ourselves at a particular point on a theoretical timeline or process.

What I think is more helpful is for us to understand what our bodies are experiencing. We can learn about hormone levels and what less estrogen means to our hearts, bones, brains, and sexual health after menopause. By listening to our bodies and staying attuned to the transition, we can grow healthy relationships with people who will understand, like close women friends and a menopause care provider. If we do so, we can make smart choices to manage or adapt to the changes in our bodies as they present themselves.

THE RATE OF CHANGE

Part of the complexity and variability of menopause is its (naturally) unpredictable pace. In fact, there is something called STRAW (the Stages of Reproductive Aging Workshop) that defines a 10-stage classification system for menopause. For our purposes, we will identify four stages of the transition into menopause and their "normal" ranges.

- ♥ Your *late reproductive years* may last as many as nine years.

- ♥ The *early menopausal transition* may last four or more years.

- ♥ The *late menopausal transition* is shorter, typically one or two years.

- ♥ *Postmenopause* is the new normal and begins after your final period.

That outline gives you a general idea of the process of change our bodies are navigating. Of course, the number of symptoms, their intensity, and their duration throughout the stages will differ depending on the individual. If skipping your period a few times or a minor change in your cycle is the only evidence you see of the transition's start, you may hardly be aware of the change. If, on the other hand, perimenopause arrives with every trick in its book, it might feel like it's dragging on forever. Both patterns are perfectly normal.

Again, for many, menopause arrives abruptly as a result of the surgical removal of ovaries, chemotherapy, radiation, premature ovarian failure, or other, preexisting conditions. For people who fall into this category, their entire experience will be determined by their age and reproductive status when these medical events occur. In general, they'll often have more challenging symptoms because of the sudden end to hormone production.

PHYSICAL CHANGES

Most of the physical changes you may observe during the menopause transition are a result of a lower level of estrogen in your system. Estrogen plays two specific roles in our bodies' physical health through the receptors I mentioned at the beginning of this chapter. First is its role in maintaining supple, healthy tissue; second is its role as a regulator.

I list the following symptoms not because you can expect to encounter them all—you may experience few; you may not notice any at all. Rather, I'm emphasizing them because many don't seem obviously related to menopause. If you understand the connection between your symptoms and menopause, you can provide important context to your health care provider to make a diagnosis. For instance, you might see a specialist to diagnose heart-related symptoms or a psychologist because you feel depressed, and they may not see menopausal patients often enough to realize there's a hormone interaction at play.

> **Dryness** is a fairly pervasive result of decreasing estrogen. You may first experience it as dry eye or dry mouth. You may assume that you need more face or body moisturizer because of age, which is true, but dryness is related to menopause, as well. Vaginal dryness occurs, too—most women experience

it starting in perimenopause and see it become more pronounced in postmenopause.

Joint pain is a commonly experienced yet rarely recognized symptom. Yes, there are estrogen receptors in your joints. That dryness that seems to occur everywhere else with menopause? We think the same thing is going on in your joints, too. It's usually described as general stiffness and achiness.

Vasomotor symptoms—hot flashes, night sweats, and flushes—are the next cluster of symptoms. They have to do with the behavior of blood vessels, which are responding to signals from the brain. If you've had migraines before, they may change in nature or disappear entirely (yes, I'll keep saying it—menopause is wildly variable). If you haven't had frequent headaches before, you might start having them now. You might also have heart palpitations, which may be associated with hot flashes but could also happen on their own.

Sleep issues are actually more common than night sweats. Many studies show that more than half of postmenopausal women experience insomnia or have difficulty falling asleep—something I've seen in my own practice. Progesterone plays a role in helping us fall and stay asleep, so declining levels cause a predictable effect. Low energy is sometimes described as a symptom of menopause transition; it may stand alone or it may result, as you'd expect, from extended sleep deprivation.

Urogenital tissues (internal and external genitals and lower urinary system) are especially vulnerable to decreased estrogen. Over the course of the menopause transition, tissues become drier and more fragile, which can lead to vaginal dryness (often an early sign); more urinary tract, bladder, and vaginal infections; and uncomfortable sex. I'll have more to say on this topic in chapter 5 (see page 76), because this particular area is where a little knowledge goes a long way.

Metabolism changes during menopause, and it's important to consciously adapt to the shift. Some of us may experience weight gain, and achy joints may make it difficult to stay active. The hair on your head may thin, and "rogue hairs" may grow in other places (such as on upper lip, chin, or eyebrow).

The best antidotes to all these symptoms are knowledge and a good sense of humor! You've managed your health (and life) so far, and you can continue to do so as these changes occur.

SELF-CARE
CHECK YOURSELF OUT—WITH A DOC

Acknowledging that every woman is unique, I'm guided by the recommendations from the American College of Obstetricians and Gynecologists (ACOG):

- An annual pelvic exam, whether or not a Pap test is due.

- A Pap screening every three to five years, depending on your age and health history.

- A mammogram every year (my recommendation) or two, starting sometime after 40 and no later than 50. An annual breast exam supplements mammograms.

- A colonoscopy or other colorectal cancer screening beginning at 50 for those with an average colon cancer risk (or 45 for African Americans, due to increased incidence and mortality rates as documented by ACOG). Your family history and genetics and the results of your first procedure will determine the frequency of subsequent screenings, which could be as infrequent as once every 10 years.

- Diabetes testing beginning at 45, with repeated testing every three years if results are normal.

- A lipid profile assessment at 45, repeated every five years.

These recommendations remain generally the same throughout life until health conditions mean you're unlikely to take action to treat something found in a screening. Eventually, we reach an age at which we wouldn't outlive a disease (a slow-growing cancer, for example) or when treatment would have a significant negative impact on our quality of life. ACOG suggests that after age 75 is a time to consider whether to continue routine screenings, especially more invasive ones.

BRAIN CHANGES

If you've ever experienced PMS symptoms—whether in yourself or in someone else—you've likely seen evidence of the connection between hormones, emotions, cognition, and mood. If your menstrual cycle gave you a short-fuse day, a weepy day, and a brain-fog day, you've had a preview of what's to come.

Moodiness or mood swings are often observed in perimenopause and can continue throughout the transition. You may feel anxious or nervous, sad, or irritable. You may have difficulty concentrating, and you may find yourself with short-term-memory lapses.

One change that can happen in both body and brain is a loss of sexual desire. If you're feeling sad or anxious, you may have less interest in sex. If you have physical changes that make sex less comfortable or less satisfying, you're likely to have less interest in it. This symptom is another instance (like with insomnia and low energy) where different aspects of menopause can feed off of or disguise one another. Checking in with yourself regularly (asking "What am I feeling now?" "What do I need now?" "What do I want now?"), in addition to journaling, can help tease apart the tangle of these issues. Chapter 5 describes more practical steps you can take for your sexual health (see pages 82 to 93).

Unfortunately, there is too little research on the brain that takes estrogen (or its absence postmenopause) into account. There's much more that we can't see and that medical researchers don't yet understand. Estrogen is believed to protect brain cell health, improve memory, and produce memory. But researchers are still trying to understand the role of estrogen in brain conditions, such as Alzheimer's disease and other forms of dementia.

Even though the research we have right now is limited, you know yourself better than anyone, and you can use your own systems and visual cues to keep your brain health on track. Again, journaling and tracking your own symptoms can be incredibly helpful here. Of course, if sadness is starting to feel like a longer-lasting depression, talk to your health care provider.

HORMONE THERAPY

When your body is no longer producing hormones, you have the option of adding them to your system. Put simply, hormone therapy provides replacement hormones to treat deficiencies. If you hear or read *HRT* (hormone replacement therapy), know that term is the older medical language for what's now called *HT*, or hormone therapy.

Hormone therapy was pretty broadly accepted around the world 20 years ago as being beneficial for menopausal women, both for daily comfort and for disease prevention. That treatment option was abruptly upended in 2002, when a long-term national health study called the Women's Health Initiative (WHI) made news headlines with the claim that HT caused breast cancer.

I well remember the summer day when that story broke. All day long, my office took calls from patients asking for advice. Normally, as a physician in a situation like this one, I would have received prior information, like studies and data to review or evaluate, before the news was reported. In this case, I did not—the study went straight to the mainstream press. That breach of process probably gave the story excessive weight, including among medical professionals.

And, as it turned out, the headlines were all wrong. The WHI finding turned out to be a statistical fluke. Subsequent analysis disproved what had been presented as stop-the-presses and stop-the-research reality. And yet, the stigma against hormone therapy remains, both among women and among health care professionals. Although every breast cancer death is a tragedy, the disease has a disproportionate presence in our decision-making. Heart disease affects many more women than breast cancer, and it currently has less effective diagnosis and treatment. At this point, 90 percent of women diagnosed with early-stage breast cancer will be cured, whereas heart disease will claim seven times more women's lives than breast cancer.

What I see in my practice is that hormone therapy benefits women's hearts, bones, brains, and sexual health as well as reduces difficult symptoms of menopause.

Quality of life is important to consider, too, as a friend realized when she found her 80-year-old mother up in a tree picking apples. My own mother would have benefited from the bone health that hormone therapy can provide. She had a hip replacement in her late 50s and never walked again; she died of complications from the surgery at age 62. My bone health, on the other hand, is still good, partly as a result of responsible hormone therapy.

HT comes in several forms: a low-dose pill or by patch, gel, skin spray, or vaginal ring. For women who have a uterus (that is, have not had a hysterectomy), the therapy is usually estrogen plus progesterone or a synthetic form of progesterone called *progestin* (EPT); progestins and progesterone protect against endometrial cancer. This therapy works best when started early in menopause and can be continued for three to five years without risk of breast cancer complications. Women who have had a hysterectomy are typically prescribed estrogen alone (ET), and risks of side effects are low even after seven years.

With every decision you make when managing your health, as in other aspects of life, you'll have to weigh risk versus benefit. Susceptibility to a number of conditions and diseases increases naturally with age. When prescribed appropriately, HT can help manage those risks. Consideration of HT for treatment of menopausal symptoms needs to be very individualized, based on each woman's current symptoms, health and family histories, and desired outcomes.

The Latest on HT

Since the WHI published its questionable conclusions in 2002, there have been ongoing controversies about hormone therapy. A few of them lend themselves to alarmist headlines, so it's vitally important to take in information through a critical lens. And interpreting research results can be a challenge—every study needs to be evaluated, considering design, scale, and potential bias. In the HT field, many studies involve meta-analysis, which means that data from multiple studies are merged to see if new insights emerge. In this method, while we're researching outcomes, we're simultaneously refining our understanding of how to prescribe hormone therapy in the first place. Problems can arise because, for example, data may have been collected on the basis of outdated forms of HT, and analysis of that data may not translate to current HT practices. Continuing analysis of WHI data released in late 2019 at the San Antonio Breast Cancer Symposium demonstrated the issue: Summaries referred to "long-term influence in breast cancer risk," but they explain that the version of HT monitored is not the same as that now in use. Today, HT is administered with micronized progesterone, so new users don't face the same risk. The WHI data confirmed a 24 percent cancer-risk reduction for women using estrogen-only HT.

In addition to my own review of studies and analysis, I follow the positions held by the North American Menopause Society (NAMS), which convenes a panel of clinicians and researchers who specialize in women's health to evaluate new evidence and update recommendations. As of this writing, NAMS says that HT is the most effective treatment for promoting sexual health, preventing bone loss, and relieving vasomotor symptoms (including hot flashes). NAMS recommends an individualized treatment plan to minimize risks and maximize benefits.

Generally speaking, if there are no factors to the contrary (such as estrogen-receptor-positive breast cancer or cardiovascular disease with known presence of plaque), I believe the benefits of HT outweigh the risks for women younger than 60 or within 10 years of their last period. If you're more than 10 years past your last period, your own personal evaluation of risks and benefits will guide you and your health care provider. The primary risk of HT later in life postmenopause is cardiovascular disease: Estrogen relaxes blood vessels, which may destabilize existing areas of plaque. If plaque is present, there is increased risk of a cardiovascular event.

Methods for delivery of HT matter, too. Transdermal estrogen, delivered through the skin rather than orally, delivers benefits without increasing the risk of stroke or thrombosis (blood clots). The general rule of HT is to maximize benefit and minimize risk, so it's important to have an individualized treatment design and take the lowest effective dose for the shortest necessary duration in order to manage symptoms.

Is HT Right for You?

Menopause is the only example in humans of endocrine failure, or organ failure, that we often choose not to treat. To me, that attitude is just not logical. I'm not sure how hormones that have been circulating through our bodies for 40 years as a critical part of our health could suddenly be considered toxic. More research is needed to clarify exactly how the role of estrogen changes as we age, so I don't have an absolute answer at this time. But I also believe that if you're 52 and have menopausal symptoms that interfere with your quality of life, two or five (or even ten or twenty) more years of hormone exposure won't be harmful, any more than if your ovaries had continued to produce hormones on their own.

Note that HT doesn't delay the symptoms of menopause—for most, it alleviates symptoms until they naturally abate over time. That amount of time is impossible to predict, which is why treatment plans need to be actively managed. Of course, some women will unfortunately have bothersome menopausal symptoms for the rest of their lives.

I understand the hesitations many women have based on media reports of a link between HT and breast cancer (a long-term consequence of the WHI's now-discredited findings). But I'm frustrated by the amount of misinformation in circulation. Current research shows that the age at which a woman reaches menopause plays a role in breast cancer risk. The risk from hormone therapy is roughly the same as the increased risk for a woman whose menopause happens five years later, because of the longer exposure to her own natural estrogen and progesterone. In this area in particular, more research is needed to tease apart some complicated interactions.

There's one risk factor I wish got more attention in the discussion around HT: having larger amounts of fat tissue during the menopause transition. Fat tissue produces estrone (a weak form of estrogen), which leads to higher overall estrogen levels. Research from the National Institutes of Health (NIH) has found that women with larger amounts of fat tissue are more likely to develop breast cancer during menopause (interestingly, the NIH also found that women with large amounts of fat tissue were less likely to develop breast cancer *before* menopause). Mentioning this risk factor is not meant to shame anyone, and I'll provide further discussion on this topic later, but it is an important medical statistic to keep in mind when considering HT.

Consider your entire health picture, including your medical history, how active you are, and your nutritional intake. A good menopause care provider can help you explore your options and risks and, if it's appropriate, prescribe the lowest effective level of the fewest possible hormones for a period of time to help you through the symptoms keeping you from living the life you'd like.

If your menopause symptoms are interfering with your life, I'd encourage you to consider all of the options open to you. With solid, evidence-based information and a supportive menopause care specialist, you're equipped to manage your own health in a way that works for you.

Alternative Therapies

Given the interest, I wish I could offer an alternative therapy as comprehensive as hormone therapy. The reality is, though, that hormones are an intrinsic part of how our bodies function for most of our lives, affecting our bones, brains, skin, and urogenital tissues. Estrogen is really a central systemic ingredient for our bodies, and except in the few circumstances I mentioned earlier, I encourage women to approach HT with an open mind. With careful planning for the elements included, the strength of the dose, the method of delivery, and the duration of therapy, hormones can work for most to ease the menopause transition without tipping the scales between risk and benefit.

However, some alternatives for individual symptoms of menopause do exist. In chapter 3, I'll share some herbal options for minimizing hot flashes. In chapter 5, I'll discuss ways to support the body and sexual health, including pharmaceutical options newly approved by the Food and Drug Administration (FDA) to address vaginal dryness, loss of desire, and painful sex as well as over-the-counter products that I find helpful. Chapter 5 will also include a number of ways to support heart health as well as bone health, including diet and some prescription drugs. Of course, a menopause care specialist should have up-to-date information on the safest and most effective alternatives to assemble a tailored course of treatment for the most bothersome symptoms.

Beyond those alternative therapies, my first recommendation, if HT is not an option, is to start taking self-care seriously as early as possible. Enter into the menopause transition at a weight healthy for your body; develop or maintain healthy exercise, nutrition, and sleep habits; and have systems in place to minimize stress. I know life sometimes throws us curveballs, but practicing self-care will give you a solid foundation for navigating what comes next. Eliminating other health concerns may make it easier to understand and address variables as they arise in menopause.

WE'RE IN THIS TOGETHER

How many women use hormone therapy after menopause? This doctor's answer: Not enough.

There's been lingering misinformation on the topic of hormone therapy since the Women's Health Initiative's 2002 headlines, which linked—inaccurately, as it turned out—hormone therapy to breast cancer. For a terrific explanation of how that research analysis went wrong, read Drs. Avrum Bluming and Carol Tavris's *Estrogen Matters: Why Taking Hormones in Menopause Improves Women's Well-Being, Lengthens Their Lives—and Doesn't Raise the Risk of Breast Cancer*.

According to data from *Estrogen Matters*, in the late 1990s, more than 40 percent of menopausal women were using hormone therapy. In 2010, it was something like 4.7 percent. More recent data, reported in 2018, focused on "symptomatic" menopausal women under 50, finding that 5 to 6 percent of that population were using hormone therapy.

In my opinion, it's long past time to reclaim HT as a treatment option, to learn everything we can about it, to lobby for continued research, to talk to each other about our experiences, and to make our own informed choices about what's right for us.

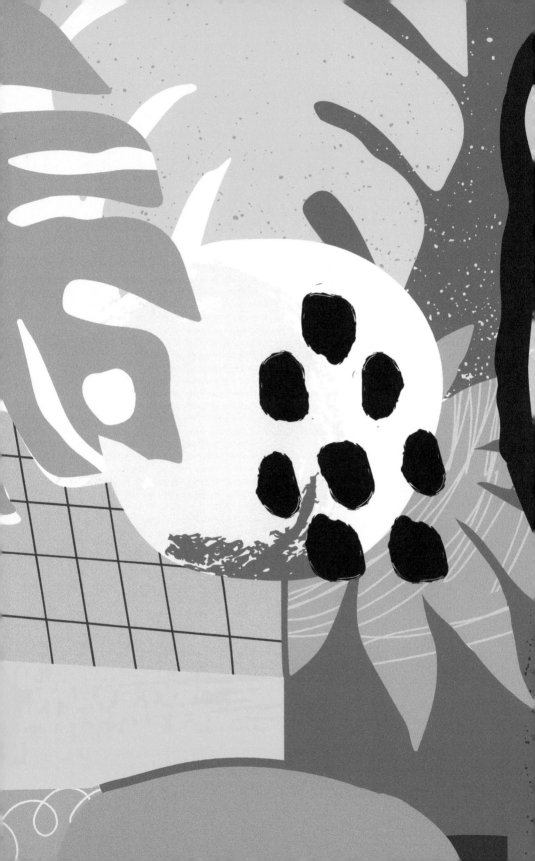

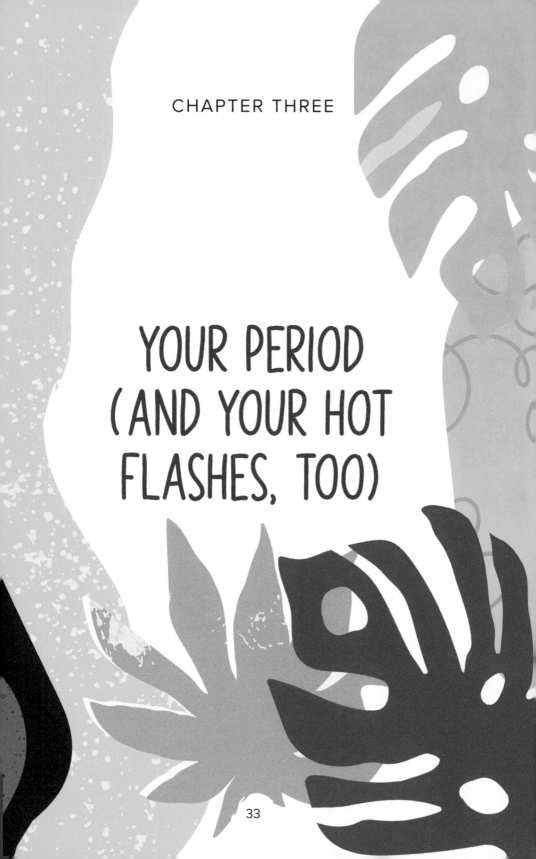

CHAPTER THREE

YOUR PERIOD (AND YOUR HOT FLASHES, TOO)

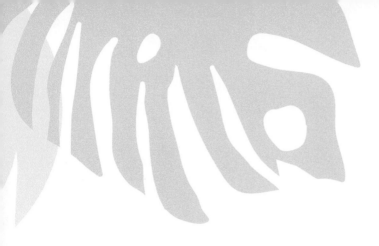

Many of us, and society at large, understand menopause by one factor: whether or not we're menstruating—which often translates to whether or not we're "of childbearing age." That complex description requires exploration by a cultural anthropologist, a psychologist, a historian, and maybe more. Because I'm a doctor, I'll talk about changes in periods and menstrual cycles as the most concrete evidence women often have that they're entering a new stage.

THE CHANGE OF "THE CHANGE"

During reproductive years, estrogen and progesterone run the show. Between the two of them, they help the uterus support a fertilized egg. A brief disruption in production of those hormones triggers our periods, during which time we shed the tissue we don't need if a pregnancy does not occur.

That much, women generally have in common. Long before we reach menopause, though, we are each on our own biological path. The general understanding is that a menstrual cycle is 28 days long, but anything shorter or longer than 7 days is also considered healthy. About a third of women have irregular periods during their reproductive years.

Remember that although the overall trend line for hormone production is down as we head toward menopause, it's not like it drops abruptly as when a faucet is turned off; it's more like a plane landing. We fluctuate; we have turbulent ups and downs as our bodies react to the slowdown by over-producing sudden spurts of hormones. The process that's been managed by the estrogen-and-progesterone partnership gets out of whack because the two hormones are no longer in sync—each is on its own path with its own timetable. It's theoretically possible for you to experience regular periods right up until your last. I've read research data that say so, but I've never seen it in my practice. What's more typical is that sometime in your 30s or 40s, you'll skip a period and thereafter will begin four to eight years of variously irregular or missing periods until you experience your last.

I want to take a moment to acknowledge, again, that for more of us than you might assume, menopause *is* like turning off a faucet. This is true, for instance, for the many women whose ovaries have been removed or damaged, whether as part of a hysterectomy, as a consequence of disease, or through injury. If you're included in this number, you have my empathy, understanding, and support. You've skipped the unpredictable years of the transition into menopause, but you've immersed very quickly into the full range of post-menopause symptoms, likely with greater intensity. Please don't hesitate to talk to your friends, family members, colleagues, and professionals about your experience, both to find support and to bring light to your story.

I'll reference again here the idea of using a health journal. Recording data about your menstrual cycle—or lack thereof—can help your health care provider in understanding your experience and determining whether there's cause for concern. How you take notes doesn't matter as much as that you do it at all. You can use a sticky note, an app on your phone, or some other method. (I wouldn't be surprised if someone out there has created a beautiful bullet journal spread for period tracking.) NAMS has an annual calendar on its website, Menopause.org; just type *menstrual calendar* in the search bar to find it. When you journal, note the dates, whether you had bleeding day by day, and whether it was heavy, typical for you, light, or spotting. Tracking over the course of a year is most helpful in identifying a monthly pattern.

Irregular Periods

If the hallmark of the beginning of the menopause transition is irregular periods, how do you know what's cause for concern? The journal tracking I described in the previous section can be used in the diagnostic process. To an extent, "irregular" is relative to what's "regular" for you (aside from some red-flag, call-your-doctor signs I'll come back to later).

As a result of hormonal fluctuations, you may find that your periods happen more often, or there may be more time in between them. Your periods may be lighter than you're used to, or they may be heavier. If you've historically had a consistent, "normal" flow—for example, two heavy days followed by two light—you could see that pattern change completely. If you've experienced clear signs of PMS—like a "menstrual migraine" or mood change—you may see those symptoms intensify or completely go away.

Keep in mind that factors that may have affected your period in the past can still overlay the hormonal changes. Those factors include the following:

- ♥ Extreme exercise

- ♥ Extreme dieting (not always deliberate—can be a result of illness)

♥ Anxiety or stress

♥ Diseases (e.g., thyroid disorders, diabetes, or sexually transmitted infections)

If you run a marathon or have a week-long flu, you might take note of it
in your menstrual calendar or health journal; it can be helpful for identifying patterns (or extraneous situations).

So, if everything is unpredictable, how do you recognize a problem?
First, trust your body. If you're accustomed to overlooking what your body
is telling you (and many of us are, as we pursue our careers, run households,
and support family and friends), take some time to tune in to yourself and
listen. You've reached a stage in life when you're more than deserving of
that time and attention.

Keep these questions in mind and call your doctor if you answer yes to
any of them:

♥ Is your flow heavier than usual, so that you're using more
than one tampon or pad per hour?

♥ Is a heavy flow accompanied by feelings of fatigue or shortness of breath? (These symptoms could signal anemia.)

♥ Have you been bleeding for more than 2 days longer than is
typical for you or for 10 or more days?

♥ Are you having periods more frequently than once every
21 days?

Heavy Periods

About a quarter of women experience heavy periods at some point in
perimenopause. The most predictable cause of unusually heavy periods
(defined as needing more than one pad or tampon per hour) during perimenopause is the fluctuation of estrogen and progesterone levels. When
estrogen is higher, periods are typically heavier; when progesterone is
higher, periods are lighter. Estrogen is a "proliferative" hormone, which

causes the lining of the uterus to thicken and grow. Progesterone is a "secretory" hormone, which causes it to shed.

Menstrual bleeding is largely directed by progesterone. What we typically experience as a consistent, two-week pulse of progesterone from ovulation during the reproductive years is now a bit of a wild card, setting our periods on a roller coaster. During menopause, the lining of the uterus changes due to less successful ovulation, leading to less progesterone, which in combination with fluctuating estrogen levels often leads to heavier periods. The irregular production of progesterone (from aging follicles) can result in more spotting leading into or following the period.

You may experience only one or two episodes of heavy flow. You may become lightheaded, so keep yourself safe. Staying hydrated and consuming enough salt can help you restore and maintain your fluid volume (I recommend soup). Adding extra iron into your diet (from foods like spinach, broccoli, legumes, turkey, red meat, and, you'll be happy to know, dark chocolate) helps produce replacement red blood cells.

If heavy periods start to become your new normal, talk to your health care provider. There is a risk of anemia, so it's a good idea to have a doctor check your blood count and iron. Depending on your test results, you may want to make changes in your diet or take nutritional supplements. You may be prescribed hormones (some version of oral contraception, like a birth control pill or IUD) to make your cycle more manageable.

With all of the above said, heavy bleeding can also be a sign of something more serious, which your health care provider should be on alert for. Polyps, fibroids, or cysts on the ovaries can cause bleeding, as can thyroid dysfunction and some medications.

I want to emphasize this: Please don't hold back when discussing your period with your health care provider. We are taught to think of periods as a secret to keep. Some patients are embarrassed to share their full experience with me, a woman gynecologist. I can imagine—and have heard from friends—that women may feel awkward sharing the "gruesome" details with their doctors. Please don't. These are natural bodily functions and nothing to be ashamed of. If you are, however, uncomfortable having this conversation with your doctor, consider speaking with a nurse practitioner in the same office or seek out a menopause care provider who you're more confident will be conversant with menopause symptoms. You deserve thorough, empathetic care!

Premature Menopause

About one in a hundred women reach natural menopause (not resulting from surgery or medical intervention) before the age of 40. Although it's possible in some cases that premature menopause is a natural transition of a woman's body, it's rare enough to suggest a medical evaluation if the cause isn't clear.

As mentioned earlier, one very clear cause of premature menopause is the **surgical removal of both ovaries**. There are a number of reasons this procedure might be done: treatment of ovarian cancer, prevention of ovarian and breast cancer in genetically high-risk women, and treatment of endometriosis or pelvic inflammatory disease. A decision to remove ovaries needs to be considered very carefully, taking into account the woman's age and the risks of using alternative treatment routes and leaving one or both ovaries in place.

Chemotherapy and radiation, both used to combat cancer cells and used individually or in combination, can damage the ovaries and make them unable to produce hormones (low-dose radiation sometimes causes only short-term damage, making recovery possible). Chemotherapy is usually "systemic," meaning it travels through the body; radiation is more site specific and therefore can be an issue if the treatment is in the pelvic area (though even then, sometimes the ovaries—or one of them—can be shielded). Rarely, the ovarian failure related to chemotherapy is temporary, and women might resume periods.

The more I study genetics, the more I recognize the enormous number of variables that we still need to understand better. **Primary ovarian insufficiency** (POI) is another category of premature menopause, the one we know the least about. POI can become apparent in women, sometimes very young or otherwise premenopausal, who stop having periods for a while or forever (for no obvious reason, like strenuous exercise regimes or eating disorders). If these women are tested for hormone levels, the results may show a high level of FSH. If a woman isn't menstruating, there is evidence that she's neither ovulating nor producing progesterone. POI is not always a complete and permanent condition. Some women will ovulate occasionally (making pregnancy possible but difficult to achieve), and others will make a full return to a normal cycle.

Premature menopause is especially challenging when it's induced by **surgery or damage**, because women experience all of the symptoms of menopause in a span of weeks or months that other women experience gradually over the course of a decade or longer. The occurrence of hot flashes, for example, is higher among women with induced menopause. The larger challenges of premature menopause are bone health, heart health, and brain health, which the medical community is starting to understand more fully. For that reason, hormone therapy is recommended for premature menopause whenever possible, starting at the onset of menopause until age 51, the median age of menopause. If hormone therapy isn't possible, it's important to assemble a set of alternative strategies to maintain bone density and heart and cognitive health.

I'm going to circle back to **surgically induced menopause**, because my conversations with patients and scanning of medical news tell me we don't have enough shared information about hysterectomies. The United States has the highest rate of hysterectomies in the world, with about 600,000 procedures a year. It's the second most common surgical procedure women receive, after C-sections. Almost 12 percent of women between 40 and 44 have a hysterectomy; by age 60, that rate is up to 30 percent, according to the National Center for Health Statistics.

I take no issue with the 10 percent of hysterectomies that are done in response to life-threatening conditions, like cancer or a uterine rupture during childbirth. I encourage health care providers and women to think twice, though, when the procedure is used as a treatment for bothersome but ultimately benign conditions, like uterine fibroids, endometriosis, heavy bleeding, and vaginal prolapse. There are other, less invasive treatments that I recommend be considered, like progestin IUDs or endometrial ablation (for heavy bleeding) or uterine artery embolectomy treatment (for fibroids).

If your health care provider recommends a hysterectomy, I urge you to ask lots of questions. Depending on the condition being treated, a hysterectomy can include only the uterus, the uterus and cervix, or the uterus, fallopian tubes, *and* ovaries. As you've learned, ovaries are vital to reproductive hormone function, so removing them sends hormone production into a tailspin. As such, it's in your interest to be especially persistent in making sure you understand why removing ovaries might be necessary as well as the risks and benefits of leaving them in place. Removing the cervix may also affect your sexual health by shortening your vagina, which I'll address in more depth in chapter 5.

Barring the presence of a gene mutation, confirmed by a reliable genetic test, that puts your ovaries or uterus at significant risk of cancer, anything from your health care provider that sounds like "While we're in there, we'll just remove x and y so there won't be a future problem" should be a red flag and an indicator for you to get a second opinion. You deserve to understand and be an active participant in decisions about your body and your health.

WE'RE IN THIS TOGETHER

If you remember when you got your first period, you might recall being "early," "late," or "right on time." That timing, of course, was in comparison to your peers, not to any objective standard.

The same applies to women at midlife. You may be in your 30s when you begin having irregular periods that signal perimenopause, or you may be in your 50s. The youngest woman I've personally encountered to have her last naturally occurring period was 39; the oldest was 60. Both of them were entirely normal, as are the majority who are closer to the median age of 51.

Furthermore, others of us have a medical or health event (like a hysterectomy) that ends our periods or induces menopause.

HOT FLASHES

Hot flashes may be the best-known symptom of menopause, and they are certainly a source of much of the humor among and about midlife women. They may start as early as perimenopause and usually before a woman's last period. Research indicates that about three-quarters of us have hot flashes to one extent or another, with enormous variation in frequency and severity.

When you have a hot flash, your skin will actually feel hot to the touch. Your skin temperature rises, and you may have an elevated heart rate or heart palpitations, which may trigger dizziness and feelings of anxiety. Your body will respond in a few ways. First, skin is likely to flush or redden, as if you ate something spicy. You may sweat as your body tries to cool off. Afterward, you may get chills. Interestingly, a small number of us actually skip the hot flash sensation and go right to chills.

Hot flashes can happen at any time of the day or night. A mild hot flash may wake you from sleep, and you may perspire heavily while sleeping, which is referred to as night sweats. For some women, night sweats are severe enough to necessitate changing bedding and clothes.

A hot flash typically lasts three to eight minutes, although depending on the situation, it may feel much longer. Four out of five women have their most disruptive hot flashes for 2 years or less; the symptoms can continue at a less perceptible level for 10 years or more. Those who experience sudden menopause as a result of surgery, disease, or injury have a higher incidence of symptoms and with more severity. According to a survey published by NAMS, African American women generally have higher rates and longer durations of hot flashes, whereas Asian American women generally experience relatively fewer; the reasons are unknown.

The Causes

We don't know everything we could about hot flashes (as is true for many other aspects of women's health). I know the data I've shared are accurate, but I can't explain them. One thing we do know is that hot flashes are related to declining estrogen. Estrogen plays a role in the thermoregulatory part of our brain, which tells our body if we are hot or cold and what to do about it. Both estrogen and progesterone are involved in regulating our vasodilation and vasoconstriction, which are the two methods through which we modify our body's temperature through skin blood flow. Vasodilation brings blood to the surface to cool us; vasoconstriction keeps the blood from the surface to conserve our body heat for vital organ function.

Once the message—"I'm hot!"—is sent by the brain, other parts of the body initiate autonomic responses that we can't control. Blood rises to the surface in an effort to cool us off, which gives us a flushed appearance. Perspiration (and subsequent chills) is another autonomic response. In a hot flash, though, the original message was entirely mistaken: We weren't too hot in the first place!

I explained in chapter 2 that as we approach menopause, estrogen and progesterone levels may fluctuate wildly. So it's logical that during menopause, a process dependent on both of these hormones—thermoregulation—would get off kilter. My hope is that further medical research gives us a clearer understanding of what each of those hormones is doing in our brains, which could set the stage for more effective treatment options. As of this writing, there are some drug trials of nonhormonal treatments, medications that influence the thermoregulatory systems to treat hot flashes (though it can take many years for drugs to make their way to market). I'm optimistic that there'll be another effective treatment option down the road, but for those who suffer the most severe hot flash symptoms, HT is, as of now, the most reliable solution.

Getting Relief

For most of us, hot flashes can be uncomfortable and inconvenient. For some of us, hot flashes are debilitating and make it hard to sleep or function normally. Aside from HT, you may be able to use other techniques to manage the frequency and intensity of hot flashes. Again, what works for someone else might not work for you—you'll need to experiment!

I think of the alternatives as falling into four categories: lifestyle, environment, stress management, and learning and avoiding triggers.

LIFESTYLE

A generally healthy lifestyle can make your hot flashes less frequent and less intense. It can also make you feel better all over while mitigating other problems, like diabetes and obesity. When I talk about a healthy lifestyle, I mean doing the following:

- Eat plenty of fresh fruits and vegetables and whole grains, and avoid processed foods and foods high in fat and added sugar.

- Engage in regular exercise—or movement of any kind—that raises your heart rate and is gentle on your joints. Aim for 60 minutes five or more days a week, though of course, start with whatever you can do, even if it seems negligible. Consider brisk walks, swimming, yoga, or tai chi.

- Maintain a healthy weight. A higher body mass index (BMI) correlates with more frequent hot flashes; eating disorders can disrupt hormones and indirectly trigger hot flashes, as well. (BMI, as a simple ratio of height to weight, is not a complete tool for individual assessment, but it is often used to aggregate data for research.)

ENVIRONMENT

Even though the hormonal changes you're experiencing have temporarily disrupted your body's temperature-regulating mechanism, you can compensate (in part) by controlling the ambient temperature. Some easy ways include the following:

- Keep the places you spend most of your time—especially where you sleep—as cool and well ventilated as possible. Your workplace may be willing to lower the thermostat to accommodate you.

- ♥ Dress in layers that you can easily add or remove. Sweat-wicking fabrics are especially helpful for layers close to your skin.

- ♥ Find a small electric fan that you can position to cool you when you need it. Look for a folding or battery-powered fan you can carry with you.

- ♥ Keep a glass or bottle of ice water nearby—if you're on the go a lot, an insulated, reusable water bottle can be an invaluable investment. When you're not drinking from it, you can use it to cool your forehead, chest, or wrists. There are also tons of products on the market that let you wear ice packs on your body.

- ♥ At night, consider cotton or specialty bedding and sleepwear products that wick moisture. If possible, you may want to keep clean, dry backup pajamas near where you sleep.

- ♥ If you have a partner, experiment with bedding that's manageable for both of you. Comforters are easy to throw off and pull back on, but more layers will allow you to personalize your side of the bed.

- ♥ Put a frozen cold pack under your pillow and turn the pillow often.

MANAGING STRESS

Several studies have linked stress with more frequent hot flashes. I've learned about stress from expert Joan Vernikos, who was a researcher and administrator at NASA's Life Sciences division from 1993 to 2000. She points out that stress alone is not a bad thing; it is a form of stimulus, and without it, life would be pretty dull. What matters is how we respond to it, and that much is within our control.

She says that we can minimize the negative aspects of stress through preparation. What that means for hot flashes is acknowledging that they may happen, understanding why they happen, and preparing practical tactics to put to use when they do. Hot flashes will still happen at inconvenient times, but it helps to have some perspective: Hot flashes aren't life-threatening, and they're usually not nearly as apparent to others as we assume they are.

Here are some simple tactics you can immediately use to put yourself in control of stress:

- ♥ Breathe. Dispel your panic by taking deep, relaxing breaths, counting to four on both the inhalation and exhalation. Try to ground yourself.

- ♥ Get up and walk around, possibly to a cooler place or to a window you can open.

- ♥ Hold a cold drink or ice pack to your face or your chest, or wet your temples or wrists.

If you have the time, look into meditation, yoga, guided relaxation, or other practices or therapies that can build your capabilities at managing your stress. Figure out your personal stress triggers and customize some tactics to help manage them in ways that work for you. In this day and age, you can find plenty of resources—many free—for stress management, like books, videos, phone apps, and guided audio meditations.

For decades, hot flashes have been accompanied—and thereby exacerbated—by embarrassment, stigma, and shame. Some of the humor on the topic can be misogynistic, reinforcing the idea that menopausal women are "out of control" or "not sexy." I hope that women can come together to support one other and reject that antiquated narrative while maintaining a sense of humor. I personally am in favor of renaming hot flashes "power surges."

IDENTIFYING TRIGGERS

Hot flashes are by their nature unpredictable. You may be able to identify patterns, though, like time of day, environment, or activities, when hot flashes are more likely. If you work to identify triggers, you can develop strategies to avoid them (and thereby hot flashes).

Some substances may trigger hot flashes. Caffeine, alcohol, and cigarettes (for some, even passive exposure to secondhand smoke) can be triggers. Hot drinks and spicy foods can be triggers, too—basically anything that might have made you a little dewy in the past. An environment or situation can also be triggering: Hot, stuffy rooms, especially when crowded, can be triggers, and so can strenuous activity, from exercise to ironing clothes or washing dishes to running to catch a train. As mentioned before, situations that raise anxiety or stress can also be triggers, which is why I recommend developing coping mechanisms you can immediately put into play.

Like everything else about menopause, hot flash triggers are unique from person to person. You may find that red wine is problematic, but white wine or beer is not. You may find that combinations of certain substances and environments are best avoided—for example, you can drink hot coffee on a cool, breezy deck but not in a small, overheated cafe. Tune in to yourself and experiment to find your own solutions.

BOTANICAL REMEDIES

I'm entirely in favor of including natural remedies in your tool kit, with a couple of points I'll encourage you to keep in mind. Just because a supplement is "natural" doesn't mean it's automatically safe. The autumn skullcap mushroom is natural—and naturally poisonous. Reliable clinical study data for herbal supplements are rare, which means you can't be certain what results to expect. Some people see great results from herbal supplements, whereas others don't (incidentally, the same may be true of a number of prescription medications). Some herbal supplements are quite potent, and some could interact with other medications you're taking or exacerbate a physical precondition. Keep these points in mind as you explore your options.

Unfortunately, botanical remedies are not subject to uniform regulations overseeing quality and effectiveness. As such, it's important to consult with a pharmacist or health care provider so you can make sure you're avoiding anything dangerous or harmful. Here are some starting points:

- ♥ Black cohosh is commonly used in Europe. A member of the buttercup family, it may be the most promising herbal treatment for hot flashes.

- ♥ Soy and red clover contain plant-based estrogen, which isn't as effective and doesn't work the same way as the estrogen synthesized for hormone treatments. Still, some women say they help.

- ♥ Vitamin E supplements have been effective for some, though scientific evidence is scant.

- ♥ Magnesium has been anecdotally reported to help with hot flashes. There is evidence to show that when taken at bedtime, magnesium may promote sleep, which may help indirectly.

I've focused on key ingredients here. If you search online for hot flash remedies, you'll find a very long list of products that may contain some of these ingredients as well as "proprietary blends" with little information about ingredients.

In nearly every clinical trial, placebos have about a 30 percent response rate. Most tested supplements recommended for menopause perform somewhat close to that rate. I don't dismiss the placebo effect, though! If taking a supplement does no harm and provides reassurance, routine, and peace of mind, I'm satisfied.

You may need to try a few options before you find what works for you. I've mentioned a journal before, and this area is another example where it may be useful. Treatment regimes, whether prescription or herbal, typically take a minimum of 30 days to show effects. Recording your symptoms and supplement use can help you determine if there's a noticeable change in your experience.

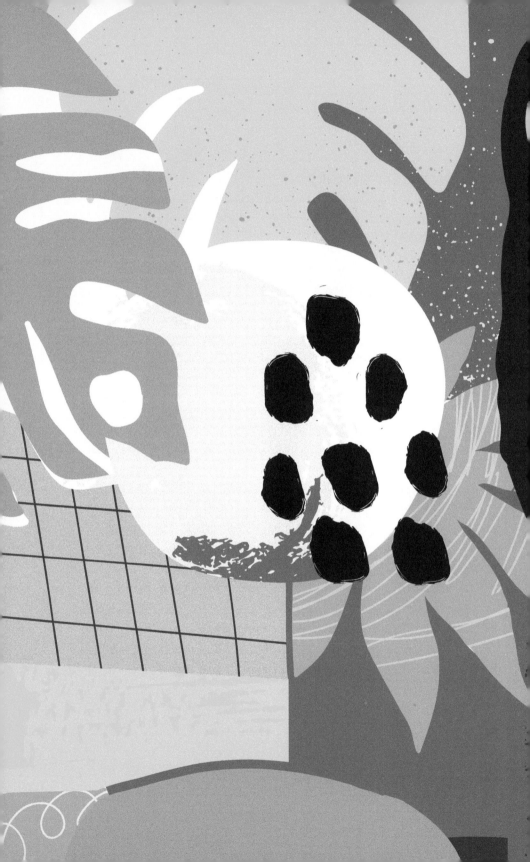

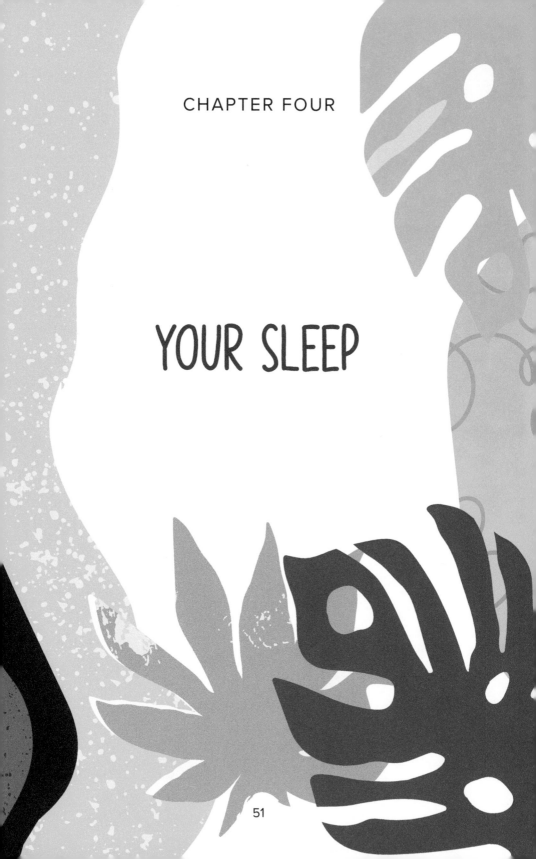

CHAPTER FOUR

YOUR SLEEP

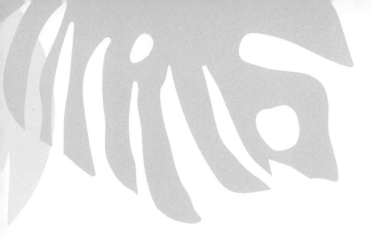

Changes in sleep patterns can begin in perimeno-pause and continue throughout the menopause transition. A lack of good sleep is one of the most common challenges that bring women to my office between regular wellness checks. The good news? Lots of people share this road, so there are plenty of strategies to experiment with to see what works for you.

SEARCHING FOR SLEEP

Sleep disruption can intersect with other conditions and events at midlife and later, so it's sometimes difficult to discern what's really a cause or an effect. You may be waiting up for kids to come home from a night out, switching jobs or considering a career change, babysitting a grandchild, contemplating continuing care for a parent, adjusting to a retired spouse, or any number of other life challenges. It's no wonder our minds spin and we find it hard to fall asleep or fall *back* asleep once we're awakened in the night!

Where Did Sleep Go?

We don't have a perfect medical explanation for why sleep disruption and insomnia are more of an issue during the stages of menopause. We do know that it's related to what we call a disruption in the HPA axis. *HPA* stands for hypothalamus, pituitary, and adrenal; *axis* is the system through which those three components work together to regulate various functions in the body. The axis is sort of the control center, sending messages to the body through hormones and neurotransmitters. When you reach for a cup of coffee, for example, neurotransmitters tell your arm muscles whether to contract or extend to do what your brain is asking. When your bladder is full, it's your brain telling you to make your way to the bathroom. In addition to fueling the HPA axis, hormones also keep neurotransmitters functioning at their peak. During menopause, there is a disruption in the HPA axis, so the control center gets out of whack, causing sleep disruption.

Progesterone, one of the hormones produced in ovaries, also functions to promote sleep. Many women see their sleep patterns change throughout their menstrual cycles even before perimenopause, suggesting that hormones do in fact influence this important function. Unsurprisingly, the changes of the menopause transition may have an even bigger impact. As progesterone levels fluctuate (beginning in perimenopause) and then decline (after menopause), you may experience intermittent—and eventually, more predictable—issues with sleep.

We know there's some change in the body's ability to regulate sleep, and that change is exacerbated by a variety of other factors, including hot flashes, which I'll discuss in the "Night Sweats" section later in this chapter (see page 58). Mood can also affect sleep, as can a number of lifestyle choices, health conditions, and external factors, like a partner's health. There's nothing like a partner with sleep apnea and restless leg syndrome—or a partner going through a menopause transition of their own—to make you dream of your own comfy bed.

Insomnia

Insomnia as a general term simply describes difficulty getting to sleep or waking in the night without being able to go back to sleep easily. Everyone has experienced a night or two of sleeplessness, like during a big move, before an important work presentation or business trip, or after a disagreement with a partner. That experience is different from an ongoing pattern of sleep disturbance. From a clinical perspective, we define chronic insomnia as a month or more with three or more days a week of interrupted sleep. But tune in to your own body to determine whether insomnia is affecting your quality of life. You may be below the clinical threshold and still feel handicapped by your fatigue.

In addition to or in combination with menopause itself, your sleep may be challenged by a number of other factors:

> An irregular schedule makes quality sleep more difficult to achieve. Sometimes our work schedules require us to change our sleep habits (I'm thinking of my health care colleagues, for example, or those who work multiple part-time jobs). Many of us must adjust our sleep to care for others on *their* irregular schedules, whether it's grandchildren who don't sleep through the night, parents who need substantial assistance, or partners who may be ill and require attention.

> I'm constantly amazed at the amount of nighttime disruption people are willing to endure for their beloved pets. It seems

that a staple of human midlife is the aging pet who needs to get up or be taken out numerous times every night—or else takes up prime real estate in the bed. Although I don't have a good solution (you may need to consult a pet trainer), I encourage you to be realistic about your priorities. Bonding with a pet is a beautiful thing, but during menopause, sleep is an important commodity. Spend your energy wisely!

This time of life may include a number of significant changes, any of which can be stressful. Remember that stress isn't inherently bad—it just signifies a challenge. Getting married can be as stressful as getting divorced; the birth of a grandchild can be as stressful as the death of a loved one; moving from one home to another can be stressful in good and bad ways at once. When stress, whether positive or negative, is high, it can be difficult to sleep. Depression and anxiety, which we'll discuss in chapter 6 (see pages 97 to 104), can cause chronic insomnia.

Our environment plays a role in the quality of our sleep—as anyone who's tried to nap in an airport can confirm. Ideally, we'd be blissfully unaware of our surroundings as we go to sleep: at a comfortable temperature, in a dark and quiet room, with a roomy bed. The reality is often starkly different. Imagine a barking dog next door, a noisy partner, or traffic outside infiltrating your environment. Even snoring, sudden movements, or trips to the bathroom can interfere with sleep.

Some medications, both prescription and over-the-counter, can interfere with sleep, as well. Cold and allergy medications, as well as medications for depression, asthma, and high blood pressure, can cause issues. Effects vary from person to person. If you notice a change in sleep when you start a new prescription, explore alternatives with your health care provider.

Health conditions other than menopause can also have an effect on your sleep. Your health care provider may call this "secondary insomnia" since it's caused by a different health condition, but it's no less of a challenge for you to overcome. If you have back or joint pain, for example, you may find it difficult to get comfortable, or you may wake up when you shift into an uncomfortable position. Sleep apnea, restless leg syndrome, and heartburn can wake you up. Breathing difficulty, whether because of a cold, allergies, asthma, or chronic pulmonary disease, will make you restless.

One last note: Your health care provider may mention "primary insomnia," which refers to insomnia that is not caused by another condition. This distinction is used to determine whether insomnia is the condition to treat or whether there's another condition that may be causing the insomnia that should be treated first. For example, if you're suffering from depression that is causing you sleeplessness, it's better to first treat the depression than the insomnia symptom.

SELF-CARE
BETTER SLEEP

There's no better time than now to devote some energy and attention to consciously designing your environment for restfulness. You deserve to be well rested, and any benefit to your sleep will pay dividends.

- Keep the place where you sleep cool.

- Eliminate as much light as you can. If you don't have a lot of control over your environment, consider a sleep mask.

- Seek out as much quiet as you can, depending on where you live. If background noise is inevitable, look into noise machines, videos, or apps to drown it out. Depending on your preference, you can find audio for "white," "pink," or "brown" noise to create a consistent sonic environment to help you sleep better.

- Whenever possible, avoid taking work to bed. Think of your bedroom as a place for restfulness and relaxation. Use your bedroom for the three Ss: sleep, sex, and sickness. If you have the flexibility and means to make your bedroom into a sanctuary, make the investment.

- Avoid screens for at least an hour before you go to bed. Screens emit blue light that interferes with melatonin production, which makes it harder to fall and stay asleep. Read a book instead!

NIGHT SWEATS

We often talk about night sweats as though they're different from hot flashes, but there's only one key difference: They happen at night. We may experience them differently—often, we're asleep, so we have less warning that they're coming. Biologically, though, it's the same event.

Causes of Night Sweats

As a form of hot flashes, night sweats result from the absence of estrogen and its impact on the thermoregulatory control area of the brain (discussed in chapter 3 in relation to hot flashes). Premenopausal women have a wide thermoregulatory zone, which allows us to adjust to temperature fluctuations and keeps us comfortable. Without estrogen, that zone becomes much narrower. Any small, even imperceptible change can move us out of that zone into unregulated body temperature: We heat up, we sweat to cool off, and we end up feeling chilled. Hot flashes also include a little burst of adrenaline, which makes a hot flash while we're sleeping especially startling—we're going from 0 to 60 in about half a minute.

Hot flashes seem to occur more frequently at night, and we're not quite sure why. It's not unusual for women to experience as many as six hot flashes in a single night—and losing that much sleep can absolutely affect your quality of life!

Strategies and Solutions for Relief

Any (or all) of the suggestions for managing hot flashes in chapter 3 can also be helpful for night sweats. I encourage my patients to invest in bedding and sleepwear that will alleviate, not exacerbate, the symptoms. I recommend cotton or sweat-wicking fabrics for both bedding and sleepwear; many synthetic materials will hold in heat and not absorb moisture. Not everyone experiences the "sweats" part of night sweats, but if you do, keep spare clothes nearby so you can quickly change without waking up more than you need to.

Keep water and a cloth near where you sleep so you can sprinkle a few drops on your face or chest or put a cold compress on your forehead and on pulse points. Consider keeping a cold pack under your pillow so you can flip the pillow for a cooldown, or invest in a pillow filled with cool gel or a cooling pad.

Because night sweats are just one of several causes of sleeplessness, consider all aspects of "sleep hygiene." If you can minimize stress, for example, you may also minimize hot flashes triggered by it. If you can boost your exercise or physical activity during the day, you can reap the benefits of better sleep and fewer triggered hot flashes. (Research shows that exercise improves sleep, though we don't know exactly why.)

Finally, antidepressants in the classes known as SSRIs and SNRIs have been shown to help sleep. *SSRI* stands for selective serotonin reuptake inhibitor, which describes how the medication works to increase serotonin in the brain. An *SNRI*, or serotonin and norepinephrine reuptake inhibitor, is used to treat anxiety in addition to depression (and some other conditions, too), which may help reduce stress that prevents restful sleep.

WE'RE IN THIS TOGETHER

The research on hot flashes and night sweats can be confusing. In numerous studies, between 75 and 80 percent of menopausal women have reported experiencing hot flashes, night sweats, or both. You might experience them for as little as two years, or they could persist for a decade (some people have them for life). Since research is often self-reported, I expect wide variation in data—after all, we all have different sensitivity to or intensity of experiences with hot flashes.

Research funded by the NIH and reported by the NAMS journal *Menopause* found four distinct patterns:

- Some women had hot flashes beginning as many as 11 years before reaching menopause, with symptoms declining after their last period.

- For some, symptoms began much closer to the final period and lasted for a longer time afterward.

- Others started experiencing hot flashes early on and continued to have symptoms with a higher frequency during menopause.

- The final pattern is the one to hope for: low symptom frequency before and during menopause.

Each individual's experience with hot flashes can be shaped by factors of health, background, and lifestyle, including race, nutrition, exercise, smoking and substance use, weight, and mental health issues, like anxiety or depression. Whatever your individual experience, know that you're not alone—nor are you without options!

STRATEGIES FOR GOOD SLEEP

Thankfully, there are plenty of resources available to help as you try out strategies to get better sleep. Here, I'll list the first steps I recommend taking, but also take a look at the Resources section (page 140) in the back of this book (and of course, consult your health care provider) for additional support.

Women's mental health expert Dr. Hadine Joffe recently presented research to the physicians of NAMS, pointing to treatment approaches effective for sleep disruption for women with hot flashes. Most of them are equally relevant for sleep generally, regardless of menopause.

> What worked best was **cognitive behavioral therapy for insomnia** (CBT-I). Cognitive behavioral therapy is psychotherapy that focuses on problem-solving by changing thought patterns or identifying counterproductive behaviors. The study didn't report why CBT-I worked so well; it may work by accelerating adaptation to new hormone patterns, or it may address midlife stresses that keep us from getting to sleep at night. It's good to know that for many, training the brain not only is possible but can be very effective!

> **Exercise** was next on the list. I recommend 60 minutes at least five days a week. If you're not currently in the habit, set a lower goal and build up from there. Get a walk in earlier in the day as opposed to later if you can—brisk exercise in the hours before bed appears to have the opposite effect, keeping you up later instead.

> **Yoga** also made the list, in third place, and as a long-time practitioner, I was happy to see it. Yoga combines the calming effect of meditation with strength training of held poses, and there are several kinds of yoga to choose from. Yoga uses breath as a form of meditation along with moving at various speeds through a series of poses. The mind-body effect of

yoga may also relieve stress and depression, both of which can interfere with sleep. As an added bonus, the breathing and meditation techniques you learn can be put to use if you do happen to wake in the night. I know yoga classes have a reputation for being pricey, but there are free and low-cost options for all skill levels, including online videos, apps, and community-based classes.

Fourth among the treatments listed was **estradiol**, mentioned in chapter 2 as a major player among estrogen hormones. Estradiol is a component of hormone therapy.

Sleep, diet, and exercise work in tandem—improvements in one bring gains to another. You're more likely to make healthy food choices when you're well rested. You'll sleep better if you've exercised (exercise has been shown to reduce anxiety and stress, which helps you sleep). It can be tempting to fixate on sleep as the one problem that needs addressing, but stepping back to look at the big picture can help us improve our sleep by taking care of our overall well-being.

Finally, sometimes old habits can work against new sleep needs. You may have to create new nighttime rituals to support self-care and good rest. An hour before bed, leave screens (and social media) behind. Try cutting out caffeine in the 8 to 12 hours before bed as well as alcohol and nicotine. Find a way to unwind to transition into the end of the day: Take a hot bath, do some journaling, or curl up with a good book. Moisturize, throw on some sweat-wicking pajamas, and tuck yourself in for a good night's sleep.

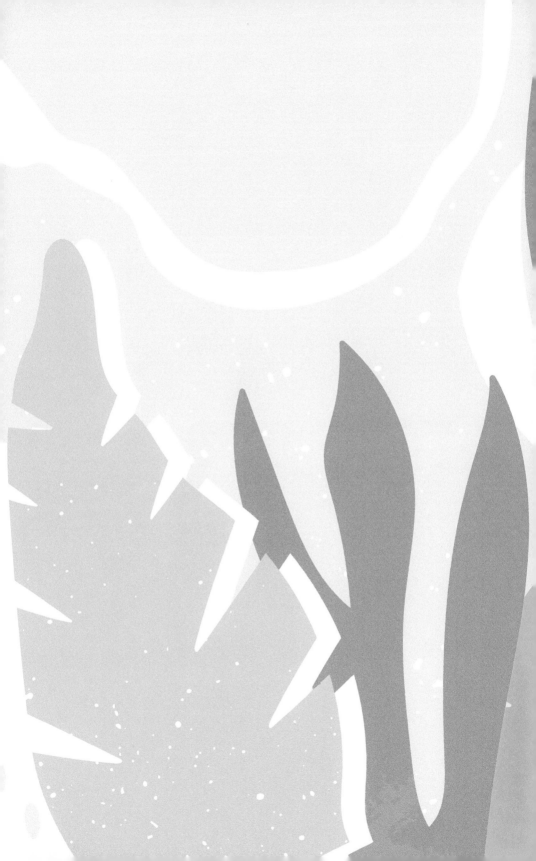

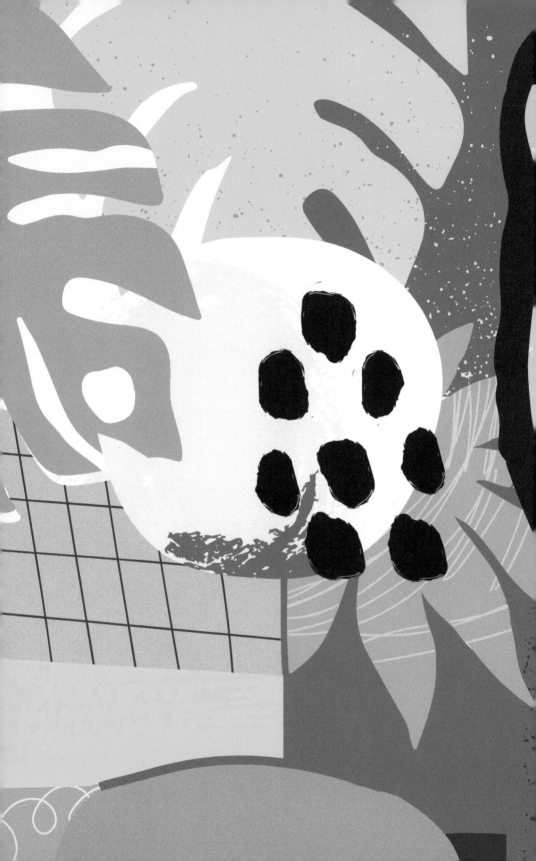

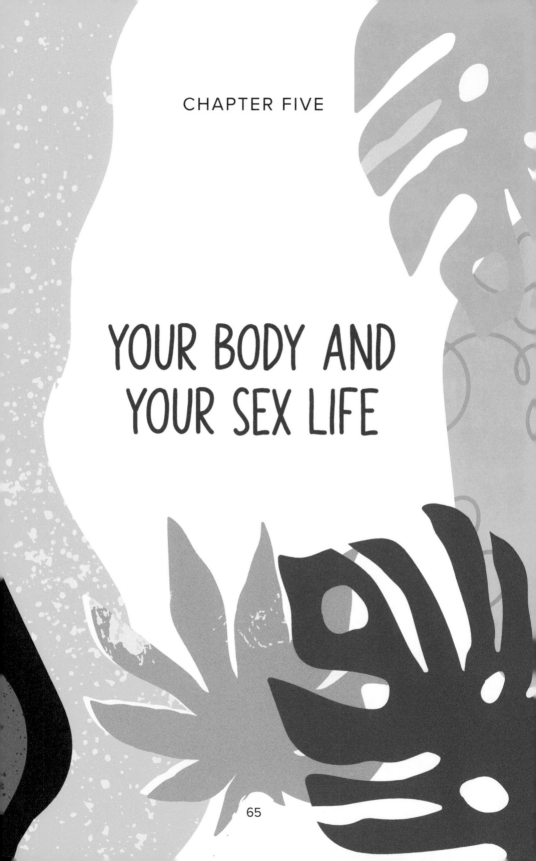

CHAPTER FIVE

YOUR BODY AND YOUR SEX LIFE

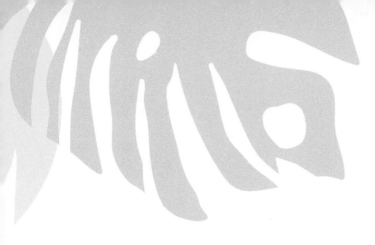

Although changes in menstrual cycles are the most obvious marker of the transition into menopause, other changes in our bodies may have a more significant impact on our lives. Understanding the physiology of menopause makes it easier to understand our experiences and what we can do to manage our health and stay on track.

BREAST HEALTH

The most important tool you have for breast health is self-awareness. You are your own personal normal. You know what your breasts look and feel like, so if there's a change, you'll notice it first.

Menopause and Your Breasts

The leading effect of menopause on breasts is actually diminishing sensation. Although we don't always think of breasts as sex organs, nipples are bundles of nerve endings that respond to touch. Some women can reach orgasm through nipple stimulation alone. For others, breast and nipple fondling is part of the "recipe" for experiencing climax. Breasts are a target organ for estrogen, so with an absence of estrogen during menopause, breasts will respond less to stimuli. As a result, you may feel less sensation.

Other changes in breasts related to menopause often include an increase in breast size. Breasts are made up of two components, fat and breast tissue. During menopause, there is increased fat deposition in the midsection, including the breasts, which results in a decrease in breast density (the ratio of breast tissue to fat). As the amount of fat increases, the density decreases, which fortunately improves the accuracy of mammogram detection of breast cancer.

Another change is that the absence of fluctuating hormone levels also tends to lead to less breast soreness during cycles. Women who have recurring cysts in their breasts may see that incidence quiet down, too.

Otherwise, breasts change with the rest of our bodies as the years pass. There's a lot of talk that associates menopause with breast cancer, but research has shown that the number one risk factor for breast cancer is actually age. Over time, we tend to accrue DNA damage, and our immune systems are less and less able to repair cells, which results in various cancers. We've also accumulated "environmental insults," like chemical exposure and unhealthy diets, that put cells at risk for cancer. That ties back to the controversy over hormone therapy and its risks and benefits (discussed in chapter 2), so I'll restate that current research shows that the risk of breast cancer associated with hormone therapy is roughly the same as the increased risk that exists if a woman's menopause happens five years later.

Solutions and Strategies for Breast Health

When we talk about breast health, we're mostly talking about preventing breast cancer. There are some threats to breast health—such as age, health history, and genetics—over which we have little to no control, and others, like nutrition and exercise, over which we do have some control.

There is a relationship between fat tissue and breast cancer. Research shows that larger amounts of body fat tissue increase the risk of developing breast cancer in postmenopausal women. Other research links obesity to cancer. The reasoning is that obesity leads to disrupted metabolic processes, causing inflammation, subsequent damage to DNA, and less efficient cellular repair (which can lead to cancers). But other related issues, like insulin and glucose levels, may be involved, as well.

A study published in the *Journal of the National Cancer Institute* late in 2019 found that "virtually any" sustained weight loss reduced breast cancer risk for women 50 and older. Women who lost about 4.5 pounds appeared to reduce their breast cancer risk by 18 percent compared with women of a similar starting weight who lost no weight. Losing 20 pounds or more reduced risk by about 32 percent.

Regular, moderate exercise can lower your risk of breast cancer. Even women who have already been diagnosed with breast cancer may improve survival rates or prevent recurrence with moderate exercise. The American Institute for Cancer Research suggests walking four or five hours a week.

The foods we eat can nurture—and maybe even protect—our bodies. Some research (though not conclusive) has demonstrated that foods that contain antioxidants may help repair wear and tear on our cells that occurs in normal everyday life. These antioxidant-rich foods, many of them fruits and vegetables, are popularly called "superfoods." Of course, there is no such thing as a miracle food, and it's most important to eat a balanced diet.

New fad diets pop up all the time. A few are evidence based and rely on science, but the vast majority are suspect. It's good to be conscious and mindful of what you're eating, but be careful about making drastic changes to your diet without basis. If you're ever in doubt, consult a professional. The following are core principles to look for when thinking about your nutrition:

♥ Eat a variety of foods. The Mediterranean diet is a great model: abundant fruits and vegetables and "good" fats (unsaturated fats, like those found in olive oil, avocados, and salmon).

♥ Avoid processed foods and foods with synthetic ingredients.

♥ Minimize fats and sugars, especially super-sweet beverages, which research has linked to increased risk of obesity as well as some forms of cancer.

♥ Eat fresh and cook your own meals when you can—doing so will give you a better sense of portion sizes and ingredients.

I often say that weight management, healthy diet, and exercise are the trifecta of good health. However, many people chasing weight management end up severely restricting their intake of nutritious calories, resulting in unhealthy, disordered eating patterns. Although sometimes resulting in weight loss, extreme dieting too often comes with a bevy of debilitating symptoms (such as bone density loss, exercise addiction, regained weight that is harder to lose the next time around, mental health conditions, or even organ failure). Although I encourage you to be mindful of your nutritional intake, I never want you to restrict yourself to the point of disordered eating. I'll discuss this further in chapter 7.

When to Check in with Your Doctor

Again, you know your breasts better than anyone. See your doctor when you notice changes, such as soreness or tenderness on one side, changes in the appearance of skin or a nipple, or a lump or mass below the skin. Self-detection remains a leading method for identifying issues early on, so your health care provider will take your concerns seriously. If you don't feel heard by your health care provider, don't give up! Speak up again or make an appointment with someone else. Your health concerns should always be taken seriously.

SELF-CARE
BREAST HEALTH

Your self-awareness and self-exams are valuable to early diagnosis. You can find good illustrated instructions for self-exams online (search for "breast self-exam how-to" or check the Resources in the back of this book, page 140).

Do a Self-Exam!

You should conduct a breast exam on yourself once a month—put a reminder on your calendar or your smartphone so you don't forget.

The first step is a visual check in the mirror, first with your arms down and then with both arms over your head. Look for any unusual, new-to-you bulges, bumps, dimpling, or puckering. Any rash or redness? Do nipples look how they usually do?

Lie on your back and use the first few fingers of the opposite hand to press lightly on your breast tissues, using a pattern that assures you're thorough. You could make circles from the nipple outward, or up and down, or whatever you choose. It's less important what the pattern is than that you're thorough and consistent.

Repeat that process of checking tissues while standing or sitting, lifting the arm you're not using over your head.

Get a Mammogram!

Self-exams are terrific, but so are mammograms! I recommend them every year starting at age 40. Take your personal health history and profile into account when setting your mammogram schedule, and keep in mind that many of the voices recommending mammograms every two years instead of annually are concerned about women dealing with false positives. But I'd rather be overly cautious than negligent: In my world, every cancer found is a cancer found early, and early diagnosis, according to *Estrogen Matters*, has led to a 90 percent survival rate for breast cancer.

OTHER CHANGES

As with breasts, sometimes it's difficult to tell what's a result of menopause and what's caused by accumulating life experiences and maturity. It's helpful, though, to be aware of what *can* be attributed to menopause. Having the big picture helps us interpret individual symptoms, understand what's short term and what may be the new normal, and choose the best routes for treatment or accommodation strategies.

Joints

My patients are often surprised when I tell them their aching joints may be a result of menopause. Osteoarthritis is the most common diagnosis (and knees are the most common site), and research is underway to better understand its relationship to hormones. What we do know is that joint cartilage is degenerating. A general trend toward dryness that affects our skin and our eyes, as we discussed in chapter 1, also has an impact on our joints, which rely on a proper balance of water and protein content to function optimally.

There are other, more serious conditions, mostly related to aging, that can cause joint discomfort. If you have joint pain that doesn't respond to lifestyle changes or acetaminophen (taken in recommended doses), tell your health care provider. If joint pain is keeping you from regular activity or from enjoying life, take a step back to evaluate changes you need to make—don't try to power through.

Eating healthy and staying active build muscle, which supports your joints and helps you feel more comfortable in your body. I'll talk more about exercise in chapter 7, but as far as your joints go, the key is to be gentle but firm in both motions and activities; swimming and tai chi are great examples. Stay in motion, whatever your abilities, and treat yourself with care and intention.

Bones

Bone is made of an outer shell and an inner network of collagen fibers called the osteoid. The osteoid builds resistance into bones, essentially letting our bones flex a bit without breaking. The outer shell is strength-ened by calcium; the osteoid is maintained by hormones.

We reach peak bone mass in our third decade, and our 30s is the ideal time to begin to be conscious of bone health. Losing bone strength is a natural process that begins from that peak (at about 30) and continues through the rest of life. Many women have lost 30 percent of their bone mass by the time they're 80. I'm going to sound repetitive here, but we can maintain bone health by eating well, including getting enough calcium, and by exercising, especially doing weight-bearing activities. Smoking and excessive alcohol consumption are as bad for bones as they are for the rest of the body. (Smoking inhibits cardiovascular health, and bones depend on healthy circulation; alcohol interferes with our ability to absorb calcium and vitamin D and interrupts cellular bone repair.)

You've probably heard that our bodies are constantly remaking themselves. For the bones, the process includes resorption (breaking down bone tissue)—"out with the old"—and formation (adding bone cells to the osteoid)—"in with the new." We want resorption and formation to stay in balance. When our bodies break down more bone than they create, we end up with osteoporosis (*osteo* means "bone" and *porosis* means "porous"), a disease that makes bones much more fragile and at risk of fracturing.

In menopause and beyond, the two-part construction of bones requires some attention. Prescription therapies for bone loss can post-pone osteoporosis for women who are at high risk of fracture and prevent further bone loss among those who already have it. Determining which medication is right for you is an important conversation to have with your health care provider. Estrogen in hormone therapy provides a fully effec-tive route for bone resilience because it feeds bone formation. Research published by the WHI indicates that estrogen significantly reduces the risk of hip fracture—by as much as 50 percent—and no treatment has been shown to better prevent osteoporosis or fractures in the spine and hips than HT.

Eyes

You may have already experienced eyesight changes or eye discomfort during your menstrual cycle, and these changes continue during menopause as a result of fluctuating hormone levels. Some women find that their contacts are a little less comfortable or that they need their readers more often. Some women report dry or irritated eyes in postmenopause, but research also shows that dry eye is also reported by women on HT.

The connection between hormones and eye function could use more research. We know that dry eye (which can cause or be caused by other symptoms) occurs more frequently as we grow older, and we know that maintaining moisture in the body overall is a priority during and after menopause.

In the meantime, I can recommend treatments. Omega-3 fatty acids, whether in fish or dietary supplements, can help. So can drinking more water, especially if you're frequently in a dry environment. There are a number of over-the-counter eye drops for replacing natural tears (make sure you get moisturizing drops, not drops aimed to reduce redness). There are prescription options for treatment, too. If you're like me, your eyesight is a critical part of what you love to do, so don't hesitate to make an appointment with an ophthalmologist if you're concerned.

Skin

The loss of moisture that comes with menopause is especially relevant to skin. With less estrogen, we have less collagen (a structural protein) and thinner skin. We lose collagen fastest during the first five years of menopause, especially if we've spent a lot of time in the sun or smoked. Prevention and treatment are most impactful earlier in the menopause transition.

Hormone changes during the menopause transition also lead some women to have a reoccurrence of acne. An imbalance of estrogen and androgen (the class of hormone that includes testosterone) is to blame. Adult acne usually requires different treatments than acne that appears during puberty (and products designed for young adults are often very drying), so if you're bothered, talk to your health care provider.

Keep yourself in your best, most radiant shape by

♥ Avoiding smoking and secondhand smoke

♥ Using a sunscreen of SPF 15 or higher when outdoors

♥ Hydrating

♥ Avoiding very hot baths or showers and drying soap products

♥ Applying moisturizing oils or lotions all over your body

I want to emphasize that last point: Lotions and oils may seem like a luxury, but you absolutely deserve to take care of yourself. Your skin is your body's largest organ, capable of receiving all kinds of information and pleasure for the rest of your body. Treat it well.

Heart Health

I interviewed Dr. Avrum Bluming, coauthor of *Estrogen Matters*, for an episode of my podcast, *The Fullness of Midlife*, and he shared some attention-getting numbers: "Heart disease kills seven times as many women in this country as breast cancer does. In every decade of a woman's life from age 40 on, heart disease is responsible for more deaths than breast cancer among women. Heart disease is responsible for more deaths than the next 15 causes of death in the United States among women."

For too long, research into the cardiovascular system and disease included mostly men as subjects, assuming that women were identical to men, just smaller. The reality is that estrogen plays a major role in women's heart health—a stark difference from men's heart health. We need more research to fully understand estrogen's role in the female cardiovascular system as well as additional therapeutic options. What we know now is that estrogen

♥ Increases "good" cholesterol (HDL, or high-density lipoprotein) and decreases "bad" cholesterol (LDL, or low-density lipoprotein). In simple terms, cholesterol is a type of fat found in our blood. LDL is "bad" because it can build up on artery walls and increase the risk of heart disease. HDL is "good" because it combats the LDL to keep arteries healthy.

♥ Keeps blood vessels supple and smooth, supporting their ability to contract and dilate.

♥ Absorbs naturally occurring free-radical particles in our blood, which can otherwise cause damage to tissues and arteries.

The problematic 2002 WHI study about the link between hormone therapy and breast cancer also muddied the waters about the effects of HT on heart health. Although there are still alarmist articles in circulation, more recent research suggests that there's a window within which hormone therapy can be introduced to provide more benefit than risk. Because arteries become less elastic after menopause, hormone therapy should begin before age 60 or within 10 years of entering menopause. Within that window, hormone therapy significantly reduces coronary artery disease and overall mortality, adding three or four years to your life.

Urogenital Changes

Without estrogen, our urogenital tissues, which include the vagina, vulva, labia, and urethra, undergo some changes. We see a reduction in tissue volume; clinical scanning and imaging support estimations that in the years following menopause, we can lose up to 80 percent of our genital "volume." This change happens partly because tissues that were plump and moisturized become thinner and drier. Some of this reduction is visible and perceptible to us: The vulva and vagina get smaller, and the vagina may become shorter and narrower. Not only is tissue shrinking, but also the vagina is changing shape. I describe vaginal folds during the reproductive years as a pleated skirt: The folds, called rugae, expand immensely, giving us the capacity to have sex comfortably and give birth vaginally. As we transition into menopause, we lose those folds, making the pleated skirt look more like a pencil skirt.

Perimenopause and menopause are major disruptors of vaginal pH levels, that is, the vagina's level of acidity. Another science lesson: *pH* stands for "potential hydrogen," and it's a measure of acidity. High acid, or an acidic environment, is less friendly to infections. The opposite of acidic is basic, and basic environments are more friendly to harmful bacteria, which can lead to infection. The scale for measuring pH goes from 0 to 14, with 0 the most acidic and 14 the most basic. The normal pH of the vagina is on the acidic side, 3.5 to 5.0. There are over-the-counter test strips and probes to measure exact pH, but don't be overly concerned with knowing the number—symptoms are what count.

Our vaginal pH levels vary a bit during our reproductive years. For example, menstrual blood has a pH of 7.4. Semen has a pH of 7 to 8, so the vaginal environment becomes more basic for a bit after penetrative intercourse with an ejaculation. Douching, even when well intentioned, flushes out healthy bacteria, so it often raises pH.

Healthy vaginal pH is maintained by an abundance of healthy bacteria called lactobacilli. Disrupting their dominance (through antibiotic use, sex, douching, or menopause) is what can cause other, less desirable bacteria and yeast to overgrow and create an infection.

With menopause, we have a new normal in our vaginal pH level, and it makes us more susceptible to infection. The most common infection related to the pH change is bacterial vaginosis (or BV), caused by the bacteria *Gardnerella vaginalis*. It's mostly an inconvenience and is typically diagnosed by the presence of a milky, gray-white discharge and a fishy odor (and possibly some itching and irritation), but it can be treated effectively with an antibiotic.

But why are midlife women also more susceptible to urinary tract and bladder infections? The primary cause is the proximity of the urethra to the vagina. The urethra, rectum, and vagina are in close proximity, so bacteria that resides on the skin normally are easily transported between them through sex, wiping, and general movement in daily living. The vagina is less hostile to invading bacteria during menopause, and tissues—including those in the urethra—are more fragile. When urethral tissues are thin and fragile, they can't stop the transport of bacteria up into the bladder, often resulting in more frequent urinary tract infections.

Again, hormone therapy helps maintain tissue health (and even reverse prior damage), defending against infections. Localized estrogen treatments, administered via a cream, a tablet, gelcaps, or a ring directly to genital tissues, increases blood flow and elasticity and moisture. In recent years, there have been some new, non-estrogen prescription drugs introduced. As of this writing, there are a couple of options to support tissue health: an oral medication and a vaginal suppository. I'm hopeful that there will continue to be new pharmaceutical developments in this space.

There are some simple steps you can take, too, to minimize your risk of infection. Vaginal moisturizers, although they don't go as far as hormone therapy, can support tissue health if they're started early in menopause, before significant tissue thinning has occurred. Using a lubricant during sex will help prevent discomfort. Empty your bladder soon after sex to flush out any bacteria that happen to be introduced by hands, saliva, toys, or your partner. If you're prone to urinary tract infections that result from sex, you may find it helpful to take a dose of an oral antibiotic with sexual activity.

Looking for some good news? If you've ever suffered from fibroids or endometriosis, both tend to regress after menopause.

Pelvic Floor

The pelvic floor is something we don't think about until we need it. At this stage in our lives, it's time to pay attention! Pelvic floor muscles play a critical role in everyday body functions, like bladder and bowel control; keeping organs in place; and intensity of orgasms.

The pelvic floor is like a sling of muscle that runs across the pubic region from front to back (from the pubic bone to the tailbone) and to the hip bones on either side. It forms an intricate figure-eight shape around the vagina, urethra, and anus, controlling, supporting, and maintaining good function in those unsung but important areas.

It's also a deep muscle that works in tandem with other muscles in the back and abdomen. All these muscles have to be balanced and working harmoniously for us to be pain free and without uncomfortable symptoms, such as a bulge that signals a uterine prolapse or the more common tendency to "laugh and leak."

The pelvic floor is subjected to unique demands compared to other body parts. It literally holds organs in place, so pressure from childbirth, obesity, trauma, heavy lifting, intense coughing, and of course, simply getting older can weaken the muscle, and that supportive sling, over time.

Symptoms can appear before menopause. You may have noticed less urinary control after the birth of a child. Maybe you noticed a slackening of the "vaginal embrace" during sex. Maybe lately you're even feeling like you're sitting on a stone "down there" or have a little bulging protrusion in your vagina. Maybe you have to urinate more often or you get more urinary tract infections. Maybe sex is more painful.

We accumulate wear and tear as we live our lives, and then, as we lose estrogen during menopause, pelvic floor muscles tend to lose tone. About half of women will experience some level of incontinence or prolapse in the course of a lifetime; many will never bring it up to a medical professional. I met a woman at a conference whose mother considered herself homebound because she was embarrassed by incontinence; she had never sought medical care. Doctors are entirely familiar with these issues and are there to provide informed care for you. Never be afraid to seek medical care when you need it, especially if you're experiencing an impact on your life!

There are surgical procedures that can help with this issue, although some are controversial. According to ACOG, a third of women who have had surgery for incontinence return for a second surgery. I recommend starting with the basics of a healthy lifestyle (such as staying active, exercising, and avoiding smoking) and a regular practice of Kegel exercises, which you may have learned as part of preparation for childbirth. If not, here's a primer on Kegels:

1. First, find the right muscles. The next time you need to urinate, stop and start the flow of urine. The same muscles you use to stop the flow are the muscles you want to exercise. You can also insert one

or two fingers inside your vagina and squeeze them. When you feel your vagina tighten, you have the right muscles. Relax those muscles, then flex them again to fix them in your memory. If you have trouble finding the right muscles consistently, see number 6.

2. When you're ready to exercise, start with an empty bladder. Sit, stand, or lie down—whatever is comfortable for you.

3. Contract your muscles as though you are pulling something up and into the vagina and hold for five seconds; completely relax your muscles for five seconds. Repeat the contraction/relaxation exercise 10 times.

4. Check your focus on isolating the pelvic floor muscles. Remember to breathe, and don't flex your abdominal, thigh, or buttock muscles.

5. When you are comfortable with five-second contractions, add another second to your contraction cycles. Work your way up to 10-second contractions and 10-second rest periods.

6. Consider adding Kegel weights (balls or barbells), which are inserted into the vagina before or while performing the exercises. Weights work the same way they do for any other muscle group, helping you isolate the correct muscles and giving you an object to focus on. It's easy to feel a vaginal weight shift as you flex your muscles.

Once you've learned the basics, you can fit pelvic floor exercises into your habits in all kinds of creative ways. I use vaginal weights and have a daily routine of "Kegeling" while I do laundry. Regularly exercising and toning your pelvic floor is simple, quick, noninvasive, and incredibly effective in reversing the symptoms of incontinence and prolapse.

Pelvic floor physical therapy has a lot of potential to resolve issues, making it worthwhile to seek treatment before considering surgery. Numerous tools and techniques are used to help train and strengthen the pelvic floor. Physical therapists who do pelvic floor work use devices that use electrical stimulation to strengthen the muscles in the pelvic floor, and there are devices for home use that use the same technology. The logic of that approach is that the electrical pulse causes the muscles to contract, which builds tone in the same way that we do when we contract the muscles ourselves (by the way, orgasm, as muscle contraction, is also great for pelvic tone).

A well-toned pelvic floor also has better blood flow and nerve pathways, which supports urogenital tissue health and offers the bonus benefit of more accessible, stronger orgasms.

WE'RE IN THIS TOGETHER

Having seen and talked to hundreds of women over decades about their sexual health, I can assure you that you're not alone. If we enter menopause at a median age of 51 (in the United States), and our life expectancy is 80-plus years, we live as much as 40 percent of our lives postmenopause. Not that long ago, menopause was associated with the end of life, but it's truly a midlife experience now.

About three-quarters of women report some menopausal symptoms. The data from numerous studies consistently represent the proportion of women experiencing some symptoms of vulvovaginal atrophy (VVA; the most common being dryness) at about half. Data from 2017 in the Women's EMPOWER Survey show that of the women with VVA, nearly 60 percent experienced pain during intercourse.

Because I know there are alternatives that can make intimacy enjoyable and satisfying, I'm frustrated that a 2013 study called REVIVE says 62 percent of women aren't aware of VVA, and 44 percent of them have never discussed their VVA symptoms with their health care provider. Only 13 percent of women reported that their health care provider initiated a conversation about painful sex. Twenty-two percent didn't talk with their partner about the reality that sex had become painful for them.

According to the Centers for Disease Control and Prevention (CDC), there are 41.7 million of us in the United States alone in the menopausal age range. We can make the reality of menopause an accepted topic of conversation—and make sure that options to keep sex fulfilling are as well accepted as reading glasses, hearing aids, and walking sticks.

YOUR SEX LIFE

Just when you no longer have to worry about the complications of contraception, you find that everything you've taken for granted about sex is suddenly up for questioning! What kind of practical joke is this?

Though testosterone is often considered a male hormone, it also serves important functions in the female reproductive system. Testosterone levels also drop during menopause. With less testosterone, you may find that your libido dips. Without estrogen, you may find that sex is uncomfortable or even painful. You may find orgasms more difficult to experience and that sex overall is not as satisfying, with or without orgasm. Because there's less blood flow and less sensitivity, you may find that you need more stimulation to compensate for less overall sensation.

By reading this book, you're already taking the first step I encourage those entering menopause to take. As with other areas of your health at this new stage, understanding the big picture of what's changed helps you develop strategies for continuing to live the life you choose. Too many of the women I talk to have been surprised by what's changed, embarrassed to bring it up, and stymied about what to do.

I ask about sexual activity as part of my check-in with patients. Some of them say, "Oh, I'm done with all that." If that's a real decision, I respect it. My fear, though, is that at least a number of them are wistful about leaving their sexuality behind and would take steps to reclaim it if it weren't embarrassing or didn't make them feel awkward or incompetent. I'm reminded of a statistic I came across regarding sex in relationships, from Sheryl Kingsberg, chief of the Division of Behavioral Medicine at the University Hospitals Case Medical Center: A healthy sexual component adds 15 to 20 percent to the perceived value of a relationship; nonexistent or bad sex subtracts 50 to 70 percent from the perceived value of the relationship. When we have it, we take it for granted. When we lose it, we miss it more than we anticipate.

Our sexuality has value beyond what it contributes to our relationships and pleasure, both physically and emotionally. Sex is

- ♥ A good aerobic workout, burning about 85 calories in 30 minutes and raising heart rates.

- ♥ A good workout for your pelvic floor, which I've already described as undervalued yet critical to ongoing health.

- ♥ A stress reliever that lowers blood pressure.

- ♥ An immune booster, linked to higher levels of infection-fighting immunoglobulin A (IgA).

- ♥ A love potion, releasing five times the normal levels of oxytocin, which makes us feel bonded, generous, and trusting.

- ♥ A painkiller. Oxytocin releases endorphins into the bloodstream, lowering pain thresholds by up to half.

- ♥ An antidepressant, through the release of oxytocin, endorphins, and serotonin, which stabilizes anxiety and improves mood.

- ♥ A cardiac protective factor. A study at Queen's University in Belfast showed that regular sex, up to three times a week, could lower the risk of heart attack by half.

Beyond being good for your relationship and good for your body and mind, I personally believe that sexuality is a part of our whole selves worth maintaining. Now that contraception is no longer a concern, get to know your new and evolving sexual self. Please talk to your partner(s) about the changes so you can explore together what works and feels best now.

And while you're talking, don't be shy about telling your health care provider about what you're experiencing and any areas where you need information, support, or therapy. Medical professionals need to do better at raising the subject of sexual health and taking women's concerns seriously when they're voiced. In a study called REVEAL, only a third of women had talked to a health care provider about sexual problems, and 80 percent of those women had to bring it up themselves.

I know it can feel awkward to bring up the topic, but it's important for health care providers to know what's on your mind. Here's an outline to help you think through (and perhaps journal about) sexual health issues:

- ♥ The nature of the problem: What's the "presenting issue"? Pain with intercourse? Uncomfortable dryness? Lack of desire?

- ♥ When the problem occurs: Are there specific times or steps in a process when you see symptoms? Do you experience the problem all the time or only during some activities?

- ♥ Lifelong versus acquired: Is the problem something you've always dealt with but it's now worse? Or is it entirely new? Did it come on gradually or suddenly? What did you first notice and when?

- ♥ Contributing factors: It can be difficult to identify these factors in yourself, but spend some time reflecting. Are you depressed or anxious? Have you suffered trauma? Is there stress or discontent in your relationship? Has your lifestyle changed?

- ♥ Exacerbating and alleviating factors: What makes symptoms better? What makes symptoms worse? What have you tried thus far, if anything, and what's been the effect?

- ♥ Impact and distress: What's the impact of this problem on your health, relationship, and life? What is it that motivates you to seek help now?

Next are some issues I hear about frequently from women in my practice along with simple steps you can take to regain control.

Low Sex Drive

Low sex drive, lost libido, loss of desire: All are different ways of saying you just don't want sex the way you used to. Many women—and men, too—experience a decline in desire over the years. This diminished desire is what causes women to tell me they're "done with all that." By definition, low libido is a problem only if you say it's a problem, and you might say it's a problem because you miss sex yourself, and the feelings it gave you, or because you recognize a void in your relationship where the intimacy used to be.

It's not always easy to determine what's disrupting desire. Sometimes it's a combination of factors from among the following:

♥ The loss of both estrogen and testosterone affects libido. We have half as much testosterone, which is most closely associated with libido, at 50 as we did at our peak at age 25.

♥ Some medications, including those for treatment of cancer, depression, and hypertension, depress libido, as do some recreational drugs.

♥ Rocky relationships can lead to a disinterest in sex, which can pile on to hormonally induced loss of desire. If a relationship is abusive, physically, sexually, or emotionally, low libido is a defense mechanism.

♥ Stress, anxiety, and fatigue can all interfere with interest in sex.

♥ Body image issues, either lifelong or arising from changes to our appearance, can shut us down sexually.

If your relationship is abusive or unsafe, please take whatever action you can right away to leave it and get to a better place. If your relationship is unsatisfying, I hope you can consider couples therapy or other forms of support to regain a foundation for intimacy.

When you're ready to address your desire for desire, start with understanding that the science of human sexuality is young, and it's different for men and women—and especially for women over 40. Older models theorized that sex for both men and women happened in neat, linear stages, beginning with desire and proceeding to arousal, then orgasm, and finally, satisfaction. More recent research confirms that women are more complicated than that. We sometimes skip phases. We can have sex and be satisfied without orgasm, or we can experience orgasm without desire.

I use a model developed by Rosemary Basson, MB, FRCP, of the University of British Columbia, to explain women's sexuality, which is important to understand at this stage. A first insight related to libido is that female sexual desire is generally more responsive than spontaneous. We're more likely to respond to sexual stimuli, whether thoughts, sights, smells, or sounds, than to spark an interest in sex out of thin air.

We need to understand that it's normal that we don't always start with desire; mostly we start in a neutral status. Instead, the more sexual stimuli we receive, the more sexual we feel. My advice? Get out your planner and schedule dates for sex. Think about what you'll wear, what movie you might watch together, how the evening might transpire. Yes, completely spontaneous sex is nice, and so is spontaneity within the act of intimacy, which can happen within a time and space you've set aside for yourselves as a couple.

According to a 2016 study by Weill Cornell Medical Center, 7.4 to 12.3 percent of us (or more; desire is tricky to measure), getting back in the habit is not enough. The unromantic name for this condition is hypoactive sexual desire disorder, or HSDD. Part of the diagnosis for this condition, to give you an idea of the complexity of women's sexuality, is for women to identify that their loss of desire causes distress to their relationships. The highest incidence of HSDD, summarized as "loss of desire associated with distress," is among the age group 45 to 64, at 12.3 percent.

There are some medical therapies that may help, although we don't yet have a "silver bullet" that works for every woman (in fact, given the differences among us, we may never find one). Studies show that testosterone therapy has led to restored sexual function, including sexual fantasies and libido. Although not yet approved by the FDA, testosterone has been prescribed "off-label" for 80 years. Talk to a menopause care specialist about whether testosterone therapy is a possibility for you. You might be prescribed a fraction of the dose of an FDA-approved male product, or a compounded (custom-made) testosterone product may be an option. Because of the scarcity of data on the long-term effects of testosterone therapy, you should be closely monitored.

The past several years have seen new products from pharmaceutical companies to address HSDD. The first to be approved by the FDA is Addyi, the brand name for flibanserin. Addyi works through brain chemistry, which is a major factor that affects desire. The many other factors and how they come into play in different combinations and proportions explain, for me, why Addyi works for some but not all women.

A more recent addition in this category is called Vyleesi. Unlike Addyi, which is a pill taken daily, Vyleesi is used as desired, similar to Viagra, 45 minutes to 12 hours before sexual activity. I expect it, like Addyi, to work for some women but not all. It's administered by injection, which will put some women off, and in the clinical trials it caused nausea for some women, mostly with the first dose. It's worth noting, though, that among the women who completed the clinical trial, most chose to continue using Vyleesi to boost their desire.

Both Addyi and Vyleesi have been approved by the FDA only for use in premenopausal women, but there shouldn't be any reason they don't work effectively in postmenopausal women; this topic, too, needs further study. Like testosterone, some providers will determine a treatment is well suited for your condition, even if not FDA approved for the population you represent. In those cases, it is being used "off-label," which only means it's not [yet] approved for that application—not necessarily that it's dangerous.

Most important of all: Only you get to decide whether your libido is something you want to reawaken or if you want to accept the change as your new normal.

Vaginal Dryness

Most of us, at some point in menopause, experience vaginal dryness, whose fancy medical name is genitourinary syndrome of menopause, or GSM. As estrogen levels decline, the vaginal lining changes. It becomes more delicate and less stretchy. There's less circulation and less lubrication. Vaginal dryness is a typical first sign of vaginal thinning, when vulvovaginal tissues shorten and tighten. It's common, you're not alone, and you're not deficient. It's a perfectly natural part of living and the menopause transition.

If you're just noticing dryness, add lubricant to your intimate encounters. Lubricants can be water based, silicone, or a hybrid of the two. My patients tend to prefer silicone lubricants because they last the longest without reapplying and they seem a little bit more slippery. Water-based lubricants are most natural and are safe to use with silicone vibrators or dilators; you may need to reapply them during intimacy, but you can turn it into part of the fun. And hybrid lubricants have some of the benefits of both silicone and water-based products.

Please use products developed specifically to be used in the vagina, and check ingredients carefully. Products based on petroleum-derived oils can change your vaginal pH, increasing your susceptibility to infections. You're worth the investment in safe, high-quality products for your comfort!

A vaginal moisturizer is the next step you can take. Beyond use during intimacy, moisturizers can be inserted into the vagina on a regular basis—a new routine, just like moisturizing your face and neck. Moisturizers strengthen vaginal tissues around the clock. Always read and follow product instructions carefully. You may adjust the frequency of use as you see its effect. Every other day is typical, but you may want daily use or find sufficient relief with a twice-a-week plan.

Hormone therapy is an option for addressing dryness, since it maintains vaginal tissue health. Localized estrogen, available as a cream, ring, tablet, or gelcap, can also support vaginal health without circulating through the entire body. According to ACOG, localized estrogen has been demonstrated to be safe even for breast cancer survivors.

There are also relatively new, non-estrogen prescriptions that can help. Osphena is a selective estrogen receptor modulator, or SERM. It affects some targeted estrogen-sensitive tissues, including the vagina, adding cells to thicken fragile tissue. As is always the case, Osphena has some side effects, and it won't be helpful for everyone. Intrarosa is another prescription option, a vaginal insert that dissolves to nourish vaginal tissues. It's designed to address pain with intercourse, and my experience with it is the same as Osphena: It doesn't work for everyone, but for some, it can be life changing.

You may have heard about laser treatments for vaginal dryness, even for "vaginal rejuvenation." These laser treatments have not been FDA approved for this condition. Although they attract attention as a magical, immediate solution, I advise women to instead pursue treatments that are evidence based and clinically sound. Laser treatments haven't met that high bar yet.

I can't overstate the importance of responding to discomfort as soon as you notice it. I've heard from too many women who've been uncomfortable during sex but were reluctant to address discomfort, often for fear of disappointing their partner. If we avoid addressing discomfort, the idea of sex can become linked in our minds with discomfort or pain, leading us to postpone or avoid intimacy.

Vaginal Pain

Let me emphasize that if you have experienced pain, *please* don't avoid it—instead, have a proper pelvic exam. Despite my best efforts as a menopause care provider, I occasionally find myself treating patients by phone: calling with a yeast infection treatment into the pharmacy, followed by an antibiotic, then another yeast treatment, when in fact it's likely the issue is something else entirely. Proper treatment requires a proper diagnosis, which often cannot happen over the phone.

One of the sources of vaginal pain is a condition called vaginismus, which can lead to the pain avoidance I described. The condition is an involuntary vaginal muscle spasm that makes penetration painful or prevents it entirely. A physical exam may be challenging; even the insertion of a tampon may be too painful. Vaginismus can have either physical or psychological causes, or both, which can make treatment complicated but entirely possible. Loss of lubrication and elasticity in the vagina can contribute to the physical equation. Psychologically, it's most often a message from your brain that's intended to protect you from pain.

Treatment for vaginismus is physical therapy and occasionally requires cognitive behavior therapy. What the treatment is doing is retraining the body and the mind to accept vaginal penetration. The physical therapy may include use of dilators, cylinders of graduated sizes that can increase your comfort over time, Botox injections, and pelvic muscle therapy. The cognitive therapies may include relaxation training or pain management techniques.

Vaginismus is one of a number of causes of painful intercourse that fall under the broader term of *dyspareunia,* or genital pain. Sometimes, solutions are simple; sometimes, finding the right condition and the right treatment is a process of testing and adjusting alternatives. You can start on your own, with vaginal dilators, for example, but I encourage you to find a menopause care provider who can guide you.

Because terminology is always evolving, there are a few words you might hear used to describe pain in any part of your vulva, which includes your labia, clitoris, and vestibule: *vulvodynia, vestibulodynia,* or *vulvar vestibulitis.* The area, degree, and type of pain can vary quite a bit. Whereas vaginismus "closes the door" to penetration, vulvodynia makes it very painful to "have the door entered" with attempted penetration. I hear the words *burning* or *tearing* by women who describe the sensation. Riding a bike or wearing tight jeans can be painful. Prolonged sitting may hurt. Removing a tampon or urination may cause pain and a burning sensation.

The vulva and vagina may look entirely normal at first glance, but there are often subtle changes that only a thorough pelvic exam can diagnose. The causes aren't always easy to determine with certainty, which makes this condition one best treated by a menopause care specialist. Treatment may include topical anesthetic ointment, prescribed medications, physical therapy, or localized hormones. It may take some experimentation to find the appropriate therapy, but don't give up! Your symptoms are real, and they can be treated effectively.

If you have persistent deep pelvic pain with penetration, especially with thrusting, explore causes with your health care provider. Common causes are pelvic adhesions, which may be scar tissue from past treatments or surgeries, endometriosis, ovarian cysts, or interstitial cystitis. Deep pain is rarely caused by cancer of the pelvic organs or by uterine fibroids. But because pain during intercourse can lead to other sexual difficulties, like vaginismus, you should address it head-on with your health care provider.

Staying Sexy

You've just made it through descriptions of the things that can challenge your sexual health after menopause. I want to assure you, though, that it's entirely possible for you to be as sexy and sexually active as you choose to be, for as long as you desire. At this stage of your life, you probably know yourself better than you ever have, which can allow you more confidence, freedom, and self-love, all of which can help you make the active choice to devote attention to yourself and give yourself the life you want.

The lack of honest, respectful guidance to resources in this arena is why I started MiddlesexMD.com, which includes lots of articles about intimacy, exploration, curiosity, and fun as well as adaptations for various life stages and conditions. Sex is about pleasure. Our sexual preferences differ greatly, and what we like is highly personal. There is no definition of "normal" here. Exploring intimacy with yourself or your partner(s) should be exciting and fun. Remember your sexual health is about safety, honesty, intimacy, consent, and ultimately, satisfaction.

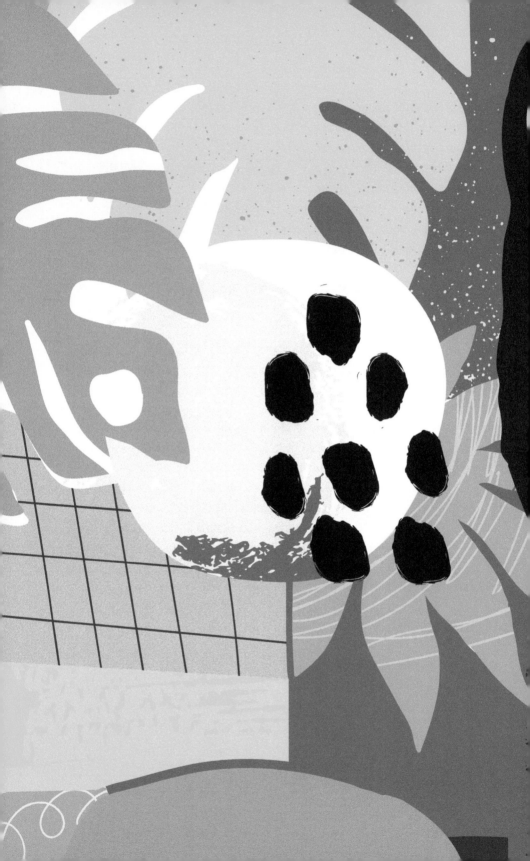

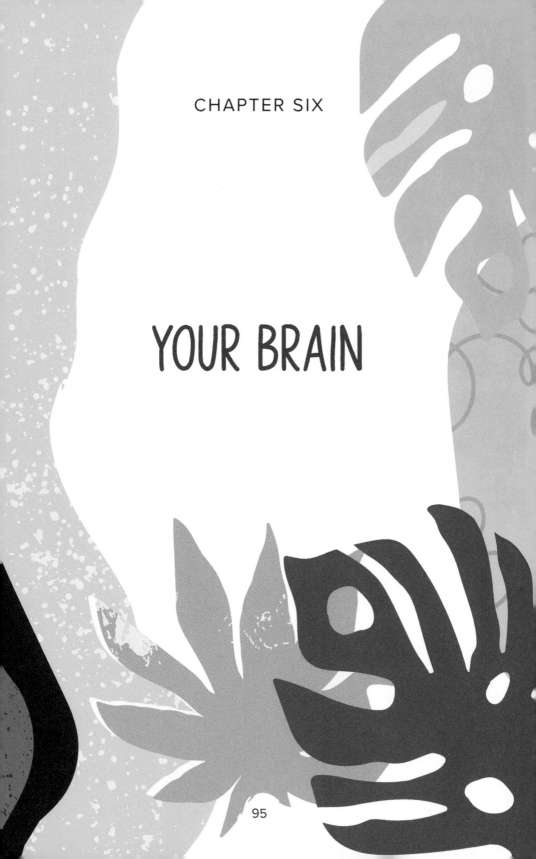

CHAPTER SIX

YOUR BRAIN

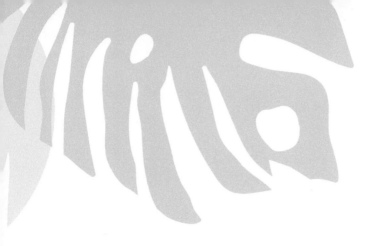

I recently heard Dr. Hadine Joffe describe the brain as an endocrine end organ or, in other words, the target for hormones. Although the brain is not traditionally included in the endocrine system, Dr. Joffe's description is functionally true: Hormones interact with areas of the brain to regulate many tissue and organ functions. We may be more familiar with the other parts of the endocrine system—like the pituitary, thyroid, and adrenal glands—but including the brain in our understanding positions us more firmly to handle emotional and intellectual changes we might experience during the menopause transition.

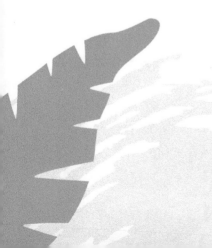

DEPRESSION

Nearly a quarter of perimenopausal and menopausal women have mood changes. We believe the cause is changes in estrogen levels, especially during periods of extreme fluctuation. If you have or had big mood changes as part of your PMS symptoms, if you've previously had a major depressive episode, or if you endured postpartum depression, you may be more susceptible to depression or other emotional issues in perimenopause.

Poor sleep quality can also affect our mental state, sometimes making us feel ineffective and out of control. An irregular menstrual cycle, which is typical during perimenopause, may also contribute to feelings of being out of control. And of course, depression can occur completely independently of menopause.

We all have sad days or frustrated days, but spending weeks or even months depressed is a different story. An extended depressive period can sometimes happen when depression builds slowly over time. Again, your health journal can be your friend and advisor. Track how you're feeling so you know when to seek help.

Screenings

There's a standard assessment for depression (called PHQ-9) that I hope your health care provider uses when you check in with them. If for some reason they don't offer it, you can take the initiative to raise the topic with answers to these questions.

How often (not at all, several days, half the days, nearly every day) in the past two weeks have you experienced any of the following?

- ♥ Little interest or pleasure in doing things

- ♥ Feeling down, depressed, or hopeless

- ♥ Trouble falling or staying asleep, or sleeping too much

- ♥ Feeling tired or having little energy

- ♥ Poor appetite or overeating

♥ Feeling bad about yourself, that you are a failure, or that you have let yourself or your family down

♥ Trouble concentrating on things, such as reading the newspaper or watching television

♥ Moving or speaking so slowly that other people could have noticed, or the opposite: being so fidgety or restless that you have been moving around a lot more than usual

♥ Thoughts that you would be better off dead or of hurting yourself in some way

How to Find Relief

The good news is that for most women, depression as part of the menopause transition is temporary; most women recover entirely.

In perimenopause, hormone therapy can help prevent major depressive episodes. Research shows that hormone therapy is especially beneficial to perimenopausal women who have both hot flashes and symptoms of depression. If you had postpartum depression or mood symptoms as part of PMS, you may want to consider asking for prophylactic (preventive) hormone therapy throughout the menopause transition. In a 2018 study published by *JAMA Psychiatry*, women on that therapy were 32 percent less likely to have symptoms of depression emerge compared to those on placebos, who were 17 percent less likely.

I talked in chapter 4 about "sleep hygiene." I can't overstate the importance of a good night's sleep—as often as possible—to minimize depressive symptoms. Sleep and depression (and anxiety, which I'll address next) can interact in a cycle: We're exhausted, so we feel less able to cope, or we're depressed, so we can't go to sleep.

I have to mention exercise again, because it has benefits in so many areas of health. There's plenty of evidence that regular exercise (and, in fact, time in nature, sometimes called "forest bathing" or "forest therapy") helps counter depression. Dr. Michael Craig Miller, a professor of psychiatry at Harvard Medical School, has found that "for some people [exercise] works as well as antidepressants, although exercise alone isn't enough for someone with severe depression."

Finally, please don't be shy about reaching out for help, especially if you're at higher risk because of previous or existing depressive diagnoses. Therapy can be helpful in many ways at any point in life but especially as you navigate this stage. You can gain not only tools for navigating depression but also ways to reshape your relationships and your self-concept to take full advantage of midlife. Your health care provider can help explore whether an antidepressant could help you break out of the cycle you're in. Therapy is a wonderful resource that can help you find appropriate solutions.

WE'RE IN THIS TOGETHER

You'll notice that therapy is recommended in response to a number of the mood-related topics in this chapter. When I meet with patients, I'm able to "read" their attitude toward therapy options and provide both explanations and resources to help them find an option that works for them. I can't do the same with readers of this book, but I can share a few things patients have found helpful.

I know some of us have received messages about therapy being in some way suspicious or the need for it being a sign of weakness. Our emotional health is as important as our physical health, and often the two are intertwined. I hope we can consider a therapist as important for mental health as a dentist is for a toothache or an ophthalmologist is for fuzzy vision.

There's a lot of variety in the therapy that's available. Consider the qualifications of the practitioner, but know that there are choices: You can participate in support groups, group therapy, or individual therapy in person or via phone or video.

Therapy doesn't have to be expensive. Some clinics offer sliding scales, you may have insurance benefits that cover mental health services, and many communities offer services through both government and nonprofit organizations.

See "Getting Support" in the Resources section of this book (page 140) for some websites that can help you locate a qualified therapist in your area. You can also ask friends or family members for recommendations. You might be surprised and affirmed to learn about their experiences with therapy. You may be part of a faith or community organization whose leaders are knowledgeable about therapists who would be a good fit for you. Your primary health care provider can offer referrals, as well. Finally, if you're embarrassed to ask personally, enlist a trusted friend to network on your behalf to locate options— and perhaps stand by you as you call for an appointment.

Finally, you don't need to reach a place of desperation before you seek help. Therapy gives you time, a structure, and a listening ear to focus on what's happening in your life.

ANXIETY

I hear many more stories of anxiety than of depression from women in my practice. My patients often reference fretting or worrying incessantly about small things. Everyday tasks—things as simple as getting the laundry done or arriving to work on time—suddenly seem challenging or difficult in new ways, even though they've been doable for 40 or more years. Many of those entering menopause fear they won't be able to find a new path at this point in their lives. Women who've been diagnosed with anxiety disorder before menopause may have a higher risk after menopause.

Role of Hormones

As with depression, we know that the variation in estrogen levels can coincide with a rise in anxiety. However, medical research has yet to identify the exact mechanism that causes it. Also like depression, anxiety can be caused by a number of factors separate from menopause, although they're happening at the same stage of life. For some of us, work can make us anxious: We may feel ourselves being sidelined from our careers or the job market because of age, or we may be switching jobs or preparing to retire. We may be facing financial stressors. We may be anxious about family as our children move farther away from home, start new jobs, or start families of their own—or if it feels like our children aren't growing up (which can cause a different kind of anxiety). Relationships and partnerships can become challenging at this stage, whether it's because we're readjusting to empty nests, friends and loved ones are dealing with illnesses, or a partner is facing a serious life change of their own. It's a time to make consequential life choices related to work, relationships, and life planning.

The point is, there are many legitimate reasons to feel anxious. Knowing that hormone fluctuations can contribute doesn't make the feeling go away—but understanding can help.

Screenings

There's a standard screening for general anxiety disorder (called GAD-7), much like the screening for depression. Again, you can take the initiative to raise the topic with answers to these questions if your health care provider doesn't.

How often (not at all, several days, half the days, nearly every day) in the past two weeks have you experienced any of the following?

- ♥ Feeling nervous, anxious, or on edge
- ♥ Not being able to stop or control worrying
- ♥ Worrying too much about different things
- ♥ Trouble relaxing
- ♥ Being so restless that it's hard to sit still
- ♥ Becoming easily annoyed or irritable
- ♥ Feeling afraid as if something awful might happen

How to Find Relief

A certain amount of anxiety is a normal part of life. But when anxiety interferes with your quality of life and day-to-day function, it's time to take action. Check in on your overall lifestyle and health habits, notably, exercise. Research shows exercise can improve mood, providing you an opportunity to refocus and regain perspective.

Beyond lifestyle, therapy is the first recommendation to treat anxiety. Cognitive behavioral therapy is typically the most effective. It is a practical form of therapy focused on problem-solving to equip you with tools to either reduce or eliminate your anxiety.

As with depression, anxiety can be mitigated with hormone therapy. If you had strong emotional swings with PMS or if you had postpartum depression, you might especially explore with your health care provider how hormone therapy might work for you.

There are also a few prescription medications for generalized anxiety disorder. Some classes of antidepressants (like the SSRIs and SNRIs mentioned for sleep in chapter 4) are helpful, as are specific antianxiety medications. As with any prescription, have a full discussion with your health care provider about risks, benefits, and possible side effects.

WE'RE IN THIS TOGETHER

NAMS reports that 23 percent of perimenopausal and post-menopausal women experience mood changes. About that same proportion have been observed to have some kind of anxiety disorder, which can include social anxiety, panic disorder, and generalized anxiety. Depression is at least twice as likely to occur for women during the menopause transition than at other times in their lives.

Hormones certainly play a part in mental health—which women who've had postpartum depression or extreme mood symptoms with PMS can attest to. It's not always clear, though, how much anxiety or depression can be attributed to other triggers or life events. Ultimately, though, the presence of anxiety or depression—regardless of cause—is enough to warrant an intervention. If depression or anxiety is getting in the way of living the life you choose for yourself, seek help. You don't have to struggle alone.

STRESS

I'll remind you here of the words of Dr. Joan Vernikos, mentioned earlier, in chapter 3: Stress is a response to a stimulus, the stimulus can be good or bad, and stress is really inherent in response to the stimulus. That is, stress isn't inherently a bad thing. The Holmes and Rahe Stress Scale, developed in 1967 by psychiatrists Thomas Holmes and Richard Rahe, lists life events—positive, negative, and neutral—that can induce stress. The list includes marriage, pregnancy, a new family member, and Christmas on one side and divorce, death of friends or family, and jail time on the other. The neutral items are life changes—in employment, residence, sleep habits, even recreation—that could be good or bad.

Stress is not only in your head. Stress, especially chronic stress, brings with it some physical health concerns, including high blood pressure, trouble with sleep, and digestive issues. But there are many things you can do to control the amount of stress you feel in response to stimuli in your life.

Why Stress Now?

Stress is not necessarily a symptom of menopause itself, but the symptoms of menopause can add stress to your life. For instance, you may be distracted wondering if you're going to get an extra-heavy period on the day of a big work event or a first date. Stress can also be a trigger for hot flashes, so ironically, just worrying about a hot flash hitting at an inopportune time can bring one on. A 2005 article in the journal *Menopause* reports that women with high levels of stress are more than five times more likely to have hot flashes.

The other answer to "why now" has to do with the number of life hurdles that intersect with midlife. We might be stressed about our parents or other family, friends, health, work, or even retirement. There's no shortage of things that can keep us awake at night if we let them.

Stress Relief Strategies

Exercise tops my list of recommendations to combat stress. Physical activity releases endorphins, which help reduce stress. When you're feeling stressed, go on a walk, do some yoga, or complete some deep-breathing exercises. These activities will all release endorphins, allowing you to feel calm so you can gain perspective on the cause of your stress.

Dr. Vernikos discusses ways we can make our responses to stress stimuli more positive than negative. The first approach is preparation, because the unknown is scarier than the known. If you have a medical procedure coming up, for example, arm yourself with information—seek out others who have had similar procedures so you know what to expect. Another approach is practice. For instance, if you find it stressful to meet up with friends or coworkers at places you haven't been before, practice using the GPS software on your phone or computer so you can visualize where you're going and how you'll get there. When you know you've mastered a skill, you don't need to be stressed about exercising it.

Mindfulness and meditation can be helpful to your stress management. From a medical perspective, prayer (private or as part of a faith group), progressive relaxation, yoga, breathing-based exercises, or any number of other practices can help calm you and deescalate your stress response. Your practice doesn't need to be elaborate or traditional, and the idea of it certainly shouldn't cause you additional stress. It's most important to find a practice that makes sense to you and that you can commit to regularly.

You may also find it helpful to see a therapist to talk through what's causing you stress. Cognitive behavioral therapy can help you identify concrete tactics to counter stress triggers. A therapist can also help you clearly identify any people or situations that might cause you stress and coach you in making changes to reduce those stressors.

Finally, there are medications that can help manage your stress responses. They are the antidepressants known as SSRIs and SNRIs, which I've also mentioned in relation to depression.

THE EMOTIONAL ROLLER COASTER

"I'm so weepy!" "I'm crying at sappy commercials!" Both are quotes I've heard from my patients in the menopause transition. Other patients of mine have found themselves extra irritable or quick to anger in a way that feels out of character for them. I emphasize "out of character" here: Some of you may be generally calm and collected; others of you may be more animated or expressive; some of you may already be managing a mood disorder. Noticing emotional changes during this stage requires self-awareness: Note what feels "normal" for you and what feels different in a way that you feel warrants attention.

Hormonal Ups and Downs

Many find the emotional roller coaster is at its worst during perimenopause, when hormone levels can fluctuate wildly from one day to the next. Again, if you experienced postpartum depression or elevated emotions during PMS, you're probably more likely to experience mood swings during perimenopause. As with depression and anxiety, the causes of mood swings are not precisely understood. We do know that they occur when estrogen is unpredictably high or low. During PMS, you may have had some warning of when the blues would hit, but the lack of a clear cycle during perimenopause may mean your emotions take you by surprise.

Mood swings can also be a secondary symptom of interrupted sleep. It's hard to maintain a cheery—or even pleasant—attitude if you're exhausted. Refer to chapter 4 to see what you might do to set yourself up to get as much restful sleep as possible.

The good news: The emotional roller coaster is a temporary ride. Since fluctuation in estrogen levels is the likely culprit, once your estrogen level reaches its "new normal," your moods will likely stabilize, too.

Mood Swing Strategies

Self-care and self-acceptance are my first recommendations for coping with mood swings. Second, exercise, sleep, and good nutrition can set you on an even keel that makes it easier to deal with the ups and downs.

Self-acceptance requires you to avoid taking either highs or lows too seriously. Know your context: Your emotions are a little off-kilter, so treat yourself with kindness. Develop strategies to help yourself regroup when emotions are high. Research shows exercise and a healthy diet can improve mood in addition to their other health benefits. Sugar and glucose spikes may only add to feelings of irritability, so a healthy, consistent diet and resisting cravings can help. Some meditation or mindfulness practice can help you pause to recognize whether you're at a high or low that's beyond your usual expectations of yourself.

For some women, hormone therapy begun during perimenopause, often in the form of low-dose contraceptives (like birth control pills) or added estradiol, can help even out estrogen levels enough to narrow the range of moods experienced. This treatment approach is not FDA approved for psychological symptoms, so talk to your doctor about your entire health history to decide whether it's right for you.

I encourage those in menopause to talk to their loved ones, and anyone they spend a lot of time with, about what they're experiencing. Mood swings can be disruptive enough on their own without adding others' hurt or mystified feelings into the mix. I had three daughters living at home when I was in perimenopause, so I'm well aware of the escalation that can happen when heightened emotions clash. Letting those around you know what you're feeling, when to take you seriously, or how to pull you back can prevent emotional collisions.

Finally, tune in to yourself (that journal writing I've described can be a great method) so that you can recognize whether you need help. Mood swings can lead us to feel unlike ourselves and out of control, which in turn can spiral into depression or anxiety. If you're feeling like you're at risk for either, or if your volatile moods are getting in the way of living your life, please reach out to your health care provider for a consultation and therapeutic options.

SELF-CARE
MINDFULNESS FOR MENTAL HEALTH

Mindfulness is a practice through which we develop the capability to be aware of the present moment without judging.

Researcher Dr. Lori Brotto recommends exercises that teach "close-focusing." Choose a single everyday object—as mundane as a raisin or a penny—and pay attention to it. This exercise reminds us that we are all capable of "focusing our dispersed minds." The next step is to apply that lesson to our lives: Choose an activity in our daily life and focus closely on it.

The goal of this practice is to achieve mindfulness: to avoid thinking only about the future or living in the past, that is, to keep our attention entirely in the present. You can choose to be mindful while cooking dinner, taking a walk, eating a meal alone or with a friend, or waiting for a bus. Focusing on the present allows us to appreciate and enjoy where we are now and thereby reduces the anxiety that can come with replaying the past or worrying about what's next.

Two of my favorite resources for further exploration are *The Miracle of Mindfulness* by Buddhist monk Thich Nhat Hanh and the CD *Mindfulness for Beginners* by University of Massachusetts Medical School professor Jon Kabat-Zinn. Both have additional books, videos, and audio widely available.

MAINTAIN YOUR BRAIN

While there isn't a cut-and-dry explanation of the biological connection between menopause and changes in memory and cognition, I've heard plenty of my patients describe "mental fog," "brain fog," or "menobrain," especially during perimenopause and early postmenopause.

It's not clear from research that hormone changes directly cause brain fog, but they're certainly behind other symptoms that affect memory and concentration. If you've ever gotten a bad night's sleep, for example, you know that you can expect your brain to operate at a less-than-optimal level. If your day is repeatedly interrupted by unpredictable hot flashes, it will be harder to maintain your focus.

Memory and cognition also change with normal aging, and hormones play a role here, as well. As we get older, blood flow to the brain may decrease and can be impacted by changes in our cardiovascular system that occur with falling estrogen levels. Our bodies also become less adept at repair over time, which affects our brain and the neural pathways we depend on for memory and cognition.

The general stresses of midlife can compound or disguise what's happening. We tend to have a lot of balls in the air at this point in our lives, whether we're caring for family or friends, managing careers, starting new relationships, or bracing ourselves for life transitions. Stress can hamper memory on its own, and it can also lead to loss of sleep.

Those who have surgically induced menopause tend to have a greater likelihood of memory issues. To counter this potential effect, hormone therapy might be considered as soon as possible after surgery.

I wish we knew more about exactly how the menopausal brain functions, especially how declining levels of estrogen affect our minds. At this point, for example, there's fascinating research underway (but no conclusive results yet) about a possible link between estrogen and Alzheimer's (and other forms of dementia). A 2013 study by the Endocrine Society showed the effect of testosterone (another hormone produced by ovaries) on memory and cognition. More research is needed that focuses specifically on women and female hormones, especially during the menopause transition.

Memory

Some disruption of short-term memory is not uncommon during perimenopause and the first few years after menopause. The good news is that, barring other age-related issues, short-term memory typically returns to its premenopause level. To deal with brain fog, develop strategies to keep track of important details, and don't beat yourself up or panic. The stress you induce by worrying unnecessarily can send you further into a foggy spiral. Note, of course, that some of us may experience this disruption in memory differently as a result of prior life experiences or a medical condition that affects focus, such as attention deficit hyperactivity disorder.

Make use of memory tricks you've learned throughout your life. Design your environment to include helpful prompts so that you can remember simple tasks. For example, designate specific spaces for your keys, wallet, phone, and glasses. Use a notebook, sticky notes, or a note on your phone to write memos for tasks or items you're worried you'll forget. I use a reminders app on my phone to record where I park my car. Try not to multitask to an unreasonable extent—be conscious about completing the task at hand before moving on to something else.

Research shows that staying active, both physically and mentally, will help your memory. Keep in touch with friends, and make a point to connect in person if you can. Try new things to stay mentally sharp, like playing new games, doing puzzles, doing crafts or finding artistic hobbies, taking classes, and reading or listening to challenging books.

By now, you know I think exercise is good for almost everything, and science backs me up on that opinion. Exercise has been shown to stimulate the growth of new brain cells and new blood vessels as well as protect the health of existing brain cells. Studies by Dr. Scott McGinnis, a neurology professor at Harvard Medical School, show a link between exercise and increased volume in the parts of the brain that control thinking and memory.

The brain relies on good circulation, which requires good heart health. Things that affect your heart health—like smoking, high cholesterol, weight, and high blood pressure—will affect your brain, as well.

Finally, have some perspective. All of us, at every age, forget something every now and then. However, if your memory lapses feel more severe and are causing you serious concern, see your health care provider to be screened. For most people, a screening will not detect cognitive impairment or dementia, which allays concerns; but if something is detected, early action can be taken.

Focus

Sometimes brain fog appears as an inability to maintain concentrated focus. A 2013 study in the journal *Menopause* described 60 percent of midlife women as reporting difficulty concentrating and other cognition issues. Again, loss of sleep or disruptive hot flashes may be causing the difficulty, but ultimately, it doesn't matter—you want to be able to focus. The digital era and the information age have added to the overload, compounding distractions that already come up with the major events of midlife.

The strategies you develop now to cope with this temporary disruption will serve you well later in life, so view this time as a practice session!

♥ Sleep is a recurring theme in countering mental fog. Revisit chapter 4 to make sure you're doing everything you can to get enough.

♥ As always, exercise. Not only is it good for your brain, but it can give you a break to calm your racing thoughts so you can concentrate on the project that matters.

♥ Try a little mindfulness before you start a project. Sit quietly for a moment and acknowledge any worries from yesterday or concerns for tomorrow that might be distracting you. Then, let go.

♥ Set a timer. I like to use an old-fashioned kitchen timer
that I twist to set. It ticks audibly and rings once the time is
up. I challenge myself to focus for 30 minutes at a time or
sometimes for 15, depending on the task and day.

♥ Take notes or doodle. For me, the doctor cliché is true—my
notes aren't very legible. But I have friends who create
written "mind maps" to help them follow a conversation
so they can recall it later.

The good news is that you can nurture your ability to focus and help it
grow. When you take all of the steps I've outlined to improve brain health,
you'll build a lasting foundation for focus as well as memory.

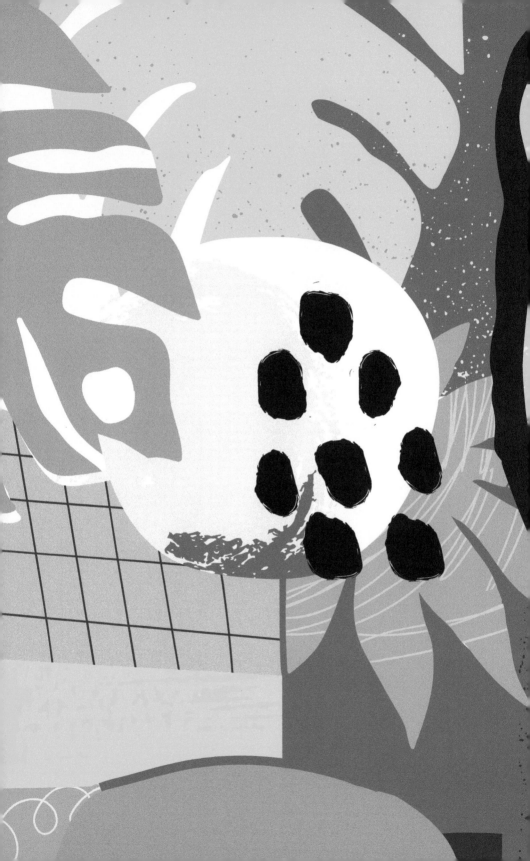

CHAPTER SEVEN

YOUR EVERYDAY HEALTH

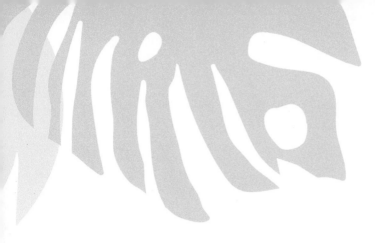

Taking the time to maintain a healthy diet and regular exercise will pay dividends not only in navigating the symptoms of menopause but also for your overall health. With your investment of time and attention, you can continue to live with spirit and confidence. In fact, these can be the healthiest years of your life!

NUTRITION

As a woman, a friend and doctor to women, and the mother of daughters, I know that our culture sends a lot of messages about how our bodies are supposed to be, about who can judge them, and about what and how much we should eat to be considered conventionally attractive and desirable. This harmful messaging often tells us it's better for us to be thin than to be healthy and, furthermore, that we need to be thin to deserve attention. This pressure comes from all angles of society, including from health care providers. I wish it weren't so.

People come in all kinds of shapes and sizes. It's just as important for us at midlife as it ever was to love ourselves and our bodies and to focus on our own happiness and health first and foremost. We're fully capable of making our own decisions about risks and benefits, effort and reward, when we're informed.

When we set intentions for our nutrition, I hope we can also be reasonable in our expectations. Knowing our own bodies is important, of course, but so is recognizing the ways the communities we live in may work against us. Some of us live in places where fresh foods are rare or expensive. Most of us are confronted with convenient, low-cost, but unhealthy food choices every day. Our families or cultures may serve traditional meals that work against our nutrition goals. And many of us are too pressed for time to think about what we're eating, let alone strategize a different approach. When we talk about nutrition, we need to be compassionate and acknowledge that some cards are just stacked against us.

I take a commonsense approach to nutrition. You need fewer calories at this stage of life. As we enter our 50s and 60s, we need about 200 fewer calories per day than we did in our 30s. Our metabolism slows during the menopause transition, so staying active becomes increasingly important. Healthy women are more likely to stay active, and they thereby maintain their health—a virtuous circle. What we're after is a balanced relationship between what we eat and how we stay active in our lives.

A Healthy Diet

I encourage my patients to focus on permanently and sustainably changing their eating habits for the long term rather than choosing a fad diet to commit to for just 8 or 12 weeks. Although rigorous calorie-counting diets can lead to weight loss, once the diet is over, old eating habits resume, and we often bounce right back to our starting weight—or even surpass it. That yo-yo effect creates long-term trauma on your body and mind. It's not a healthy state; it's better to develop a new normal that works for you on a consistent basis.

If you want a diet plan to migrate toward habit changes, I recommend the Mediterranean diet. Vegan and vegetarian diets can also be healthy and have been linked to greater longevity. The Mediterranean diet, which is considered heart healthy, is centered on vegetables, fruits, whole grains, and healthy fats. In addition to eating those foods every day, you eat fish, poultry, beans, and eggs throughout the week. Red meat is included on a limited basis.

"Healthy fats" deserve more attention, because we've been conditioned to regard fats as bad. True to the origins of the diet in Greece and Italy, in studies of cardiovascular health, olive oil, nuts, and seeds are considered healthy fats. They're sources of monounsaturated fat, which studies have found to lower overall cholesterol and, with that, "bad" (LDL) cholesterol. Fatty fish are also healthy fats in the Mediterranean diet. Salmon, lake trout, herring, albacore tuna, and others offer omega-3 fatty acids, which have heart health benefits.

Another thing I appreciate about the Mediterranean diet is that it's often described as a lifestyle rather than a regimen. Imagine gathering with friends on a sunny terrace to share bread (whole grain, of course), olives, and a glass of wine. The social aspect of eating is part of the ethos of the diet and can actually help us be more mindful and in control of our eating. Of course, we live in reality, so our version of social eating may look more like carrying our lunch to the break room at work or a quick family dinner than an hours-long meal on a sunny terrace. But those options are preferable to standing in the kitchen to wolf down a snack or binge eating late at night. The principle here is to be more conscious of where, when, and what you're eating. Start small: See if you can add one or two more leisurely or mindful dining experiences to your week.

I can't talk about a healthy diet without acknowledging that midlife can be a high-risk time for developing (or redeveloping) an eating disorder. The National Association of Anorexia Nervosa and Associated Disorders says that more than 10 percent of women over 50 engage in eating-disorder behaviors.

Adolescence and perimenopause share a few similarities that may explain this behavior: Both are transitions to a new stage of life, about which we may feel some stress or ambivalence. In both cases, our bodies are changing in ways we may or may not like, beyond our control. Estrogen has been identified as having a possible role in triggering adolescent eating disorders, which suggests it may be at play in midlife disorders, too, though more research is needed.

If you have an eating disorder or had one earlier in life, or if you're experiencing an event that's making you feel especially lonely or powerless, like the loss of a partner, you may be susceptible to disordered eating patterns during menopause. Talk to a health care professional as soon as you suspect that you (or someone you care about) may have an eating disorder. At midlife, our bodies are less resilient, and eating disorders can affect bone density, the kidneys, and the heart.

Our goal is a healthy diet, one that enhances our overall health with essential nutrition.

Strategies for a Balanced Diet

If you're looking to shift to a different way of eating—one that you can maintain—I encourage taking things a step at a time. Choose a tactic to implement this week or month, and add to it as you're ready. That approach will help you adapt to a new eating plan rather than view it as a restrictive or difficult diet.

Portion size is a place to start. It helps to have visual reference points, and measuring portion sizes based on sight is much less tedious than counting calories. (Some people find calorie-counting programs to be useful. However, if calorie counting becomes an obstacle to mindful eating or triggers disordered eating behaviors, don't do it!) Any approach that is sustainable and supports healthy eating is positive. Consider the following size equivalents to help guide you:

- ♥ For meat or poultry, visualize a deck of playing cards.

- ♥ A half of a baseball is about the size of a healthy serving of cooked grains or pasta.

- ♥ A standard light bulb represents the size of a serving of a fruit or vegetable.

- ♥ For estimating cheese, visualize a set of four dice.

Next, take on menu planning. The traditional American diet is typically centered on meat, whereas the Mediterranean diet, although it may include meat, is designed more around vegetables. While rethinking menu design, consider ways to replace red meat with other, more healthy options. Poultry and beans can provide protein, and you can feature fish or seafood a couple of times a week.

Within that framework of menu plans, try tackling these tips one at a time:

- ♥ Add a serving of fruit or vegetables to every meal, and stock up for snacks. The goal is 7 to 10 servings of fruits and vegetables every day. Raw is better than cooked, generally speaking.

- ♥ Develop a nut habit when snacking. Almonds, pistachios, walnuts, and cashews are tasty, have staying power, and fall into the "healthy fat" category.

- ♥ Swap out butter for olive oil. Whether for cooking or eating, it's a healthier option.

- ♥ Up your hydration. This healthy habit can include reaching for a drink of water or herbal tea instead of a candy bar when hitting a lull, but it can also mean snacking on a juicy peach or some cucumber slices.

- ♥ Experiment with spices and herbs to replace heavy sauces, butter, or salt.

- ♥ Try different cooking methods. Grilling, for example, is a healthier preparation for fish than breading and frying.

- ♥ Shift to whole-grain versions of foods you love, whether pasta, bread, crackers, or cereal. Eat a variety of grains, like farro, barley, quinoa, and millet, that offer protein and complex carbohydrates.

In my conversations with those in menopause, the number one obstacle I hear related to changing eating habits is objection from partners. For many of us, finicky children are no longer at the dinner table, but a partner may not want to eat "nuts and berries," or they may have family-favorite recipes that they're unhappy about giving up. I don't have a perfect solution for that obstacle, but I'll tell you one thing: Your health (and feeling good about yourself) is important. Start by taking control of what you can—your breakfast, your lunch, your snacks, your portion size—while you figure out the bigger picture.

Diet and a Shifting Shape

Weight gain itself is more likely a result of aging and lifestyle changes than menopause (or HT). What menopause may do is change our body shapes. At this stage, women typically store more belly fat—visceral fat in the abdomen. Belly fat makes us wider around the waist as opposed to the hips.

Unfortunately, belly fat is linked to cardiovascular disease, type 2 diabetes, high blood pressure, and other health problems. Fortunately, it responds to the same healthy habits you want to develop for your overall health and wellness:

- ♥ Match your food intake to your activity level, concentrating on foods with lower calories and higher nutrient levels, like fresh fruits and vegetables. Speaking in a very general sense for postmenopausal women, 1,600 calories is a good target to maintain—but again, this number will vary with your lifestyle. For example, if you're an extreme athlete, you can consume more; if you're more sedentary, consume fewer.

- ♥ Exercise regularly.

- ♥ Manage stress. Exhaustion and stress make it more difficult to eat well and exercise.

Alcohol

I'm a fan of a glass of wine with friends or at the end of a particularly challenging day. I think we need to be aware, though, that like so much of the rest of life, there are risks and benefits. I heard Dr. Connie Newman, of the New York University School of Medicine, give a presentation with the subtitle, "A Sobering Issue." She reported that the early 2000s to the mid-2010s saw an 84 percent increase in alcohol use among women. The largest increase was among 55-to-64-year-olds.

I'm sure many of us can relate, as Dr. Newman described, to thinking "it's the remedy for a stressful week." Alcohol is relaxing. It's social. But it's good to be aware that there can be a subtle shift from use to overuse.

As women age, alcohol affects them more. Women's bodies hold less water and have higher body fat, so it takes relatively lower amounts of alcohol for women (compared to men) to see some negative effects. Alcohol can also be a trigger for hot flashes, which, as described in chapter 3, can interfere with sleep, increase stress, and thereby spur more drinking. Alcoholic beverages also carry calories: Even a glass of red wine can pack up to 200 calories, which is over one-tenth of the daily budget for a typical midlife woman.

There are health effects, of course, from overconsumption. According to the 2019 NAMS meeting, there is a 10 to 12 percent increase in risk of breast cancer for women who consume one serving of alcohol each day. For women who are having two to four servings a day, that risk may be increased by 40 to 50 percent above their baseline risk.

SELF-CARE
HYDRATION FOR HEALTH

It's especially important at this stage to stay hydrated, because your body (bones, joints, muscles, skin) holds less water. Carrying a water bottle—and drinking from it—is great, but I like the concepts in Dr. Dana Cohen's book, *Quench: Beat Fatigue, Drop Weight, and Heal Your Body through the New Science of Optimum Hydration*. Try some of these options, in addition to, of course, drinking water:

- The top five hydrating fruits are star fruit, watermelon, strawberries, grapefruit, and cantaloupe. Keep them on hand whenever they're available as delicious, fresh snacks or meal add-ons.

- The top five hydrating vegetables are cucumbers, romaine lettuce, celery, radishes, and zucchini. Most are good for snacks, and they can be combined for a lunchtime salad.

- Smoothies are easy to make and tailor to the season and time of day. Recipes are readily available; be aware of the calories that can sneak in. One of my favorites is made with cucumber, watermelon, and water.

- Frozen fruits (like grapes) can be a satisfying—and hydrating—snack. Grown-up popsicles made with puréed fruit (and leftover smoothies) can be part of a postexercise cooldown.

Keep in mind that alcohol and caffeine are diuretics—they don't support hydration.

EXERCISE

You may have noticed a recurring theme throughout this book: the importance of exercise. I mention it not only because of theoretical health benefits but because regular activity is key to living a full, rich life. That tenet holds true whether we are walking a dog, hiking the Alps, shopping for groceries, keeping up with our grandchildren, volunteering at a work or community event, running or walking a 5K, going to physical therapy appointments, swimming in a pool, or making gardening dreams a reality.

The Benefits

As discussed throughout this book, exercise can help mitigate several effects of menopause: It is linked to a decrease in hot flashes, it promotes restful sleep, it can aid in managing stress (another trigger for hot flashes), and it can reduce symptoms of depression and anxiety. And, of course, it burns calories, which helps us manage changes in metabolism and weight distribution that occur with menopause.

Evidence shows that exercise may also help prevent several chronic illnesses that come with aging. Longitudinal studies have found that people who are more fit at midlife have lower levels of chronic illnesses, like heart failure, diabetes, Alzheimer's disease, and colon and lung cancers, as they age. Although other factors, such as heredity, play a role, in general, higher fitness levels were strongly linked with lower rates of major chronic illnesses and "compression of morbidity"—meaning that debilitating illness doesn't happen until close to the end of life.

I can also tell you from my own personal experience that a regular, moderately challenging exercise regimen reduces the aches and pains associated with aging. It helps provide support to make it possible to keep up with normal activities of daily life. It provides regulation, from mood to bowel function. If you feel stronger and more physically capable, you will feel capable and in control of your life.

How Much? How Often?

Let me encourage you to start where you are. If you're not currently exercising at all, start with a 10-minute walk three times a week around the neighborhood after dinner. Once you've built that habit, you can extend it when you're ready.

As with nutrition, you're looking to form sustainable habits—so don't rush into an overly ambitious new exercise regime! You'll likely be too sore to keep it up, and you risk injury that will sideline you while you recover. (Of course, always see your doctor before you start a strenuous new workout regime.) If you already exercise regularly, consider mixing it up to give your body different workouts.

Let's talk about what kinds of exercise are part of a healthy routine at midlife:

♥ **Cardio** is the aerobic activity that gets your heart rate up. If you're walking, it's walking fast enough so you can talk but not sing, about three-and-a-half miles per hour. Biking, swimming, and dancing can also be aerobic, which means Zumba and comparable group workouts count—or you can go dancing with friends.

♥ **Strength training** helps maintain muscle tone at a time when you're naturally losing muscle mass. Weights, resistance bands, exercise machines, or your own body weight can be a part of the activity. When thinking about muscle tone, I encourage women to think not just about arms and legs but also about their core, which makes Pilates a good option. A strong core supports balance, and it prevents back pain, too. And while we're at it, let's consider the pelvic floor. Chapter 5 discusses the important jobs our pelvic floors do, and Kegel exercises are a legitimate and important part of your overall exercise routine.

♥ **Flexibility** is maintained through stretching and toning. You'll experience the benefits in range of motion, and stretching is also promoting the internal health of tendons and joints. I'm a very big fan of yoga, which has been very helpful to me in maintaining flexibility and in managing stress. Bonus: It also maintains muscle strength.

♥ **Balance** is another aspect of our physical health that can diminish as we age; injuries from falls can be especially damaging if we're losing bone mass and tensile strength, the attribute that lets our bones bend without breaking. Fortunately, balance is entirely responsive to practice. Tai chi is an excellent discipline for improving balance, and yoga—or just a few yoga poses—can be, too. You can develop your own simple practice, as well, like standing on one foot, without aid, for 10 seconds, followed by shifting from standing on your toes to standing on your heels.

You are worthy of time for yourself, and it's important to make movement a priority. You can readily find books, videos, and websites that can coach you through a new routine wherever you are, if you'd like to go it alone. If you find it helpful to enroll in a class or join or form a group to boost your habit making, try it out! Having a friend or two with you can make it fun and hold you accountable, and many communities offer low-cost options through a YMCA, hospital, school, or other organization.

The CDC recommends two-and-a-half hours of aerobic exercise every week, which translates into half an hour five days a week. I know that for many of us it sounds ambitious, but I really view that much exercise as a minimum to work toward. The CDC also recommends strength training two days a week. I personally recommend doing Kegel exercises daily—I find that doing them daily makes it easier to maintain the habit. I add balance exercises to my Kegels if I'm not also doing yoga.

The components I listed can be used to create a routine that works for you. If you do yoga twice a week, you're addressing both balance and flexibility; plan for some cardio, as well (my bicycle is my best friend all summer). If you're a Zumba fan, you're getting cardio and strength-training workouts at the same time; take a few walks on the days you don't have class. If you have a chronic condition or disability that limits or prevents physical activity, your health care provider or physical therapist can help you determine what might be possible for you, either on your own or with assistance. Again, starting where you are and adding increments of motion as you're able will support your overall health.

If what I'm describing is far from your current reality, don't despair! Although I absolutely encourage women to understand that their bodies both need and want attention, I also know that habits and routines take time to build and take hold. I think of James Clear's advice in the early chapters of *Atomic Habits: An Easy and Proven Way to Build Good Habits and Break Bad Ones*: If you can make each day just 1 percent more active than the day before, by the end of six months, you'll have substantially improved your health!

Advice for Athletes (and Couch Potatoes, Too!)

Whatever you choose to do, and however enthusiastically, please listen to and understand your body. Once again, a journal can help map possible connections between what you're doing and how you're feeling. I'm confident that you'll almost always see positive correlations between exercise and sleep, exercise and mood, and exercise and healthy food choices.

You may also, though, see some evidence that you're causing some physical stress. The top issues I see are injuries that result from overuse. Keep in mind that your joints aren't as "juicy" as they used to be, and tissues aren't quite as elastic. Warm up conscientiously before doing strenuous activities, and take some time for a stretching cooldown, too. Honor your body by moving with deliberation, without bouncing or jerking while stretching—hold positions instead of moving frenetically. Having good form is extremely important and can prevent serious injury. If you're unsure, ask a coach or some kind of professional.

If something hurts, don't do it. I wish the phrase "no pain, no gain" did not exist. It discourages us from identifying the boundary between pleasantly sore muscles and an injury that requires rest or even medical attention.

Speaking of medical attention, the kind of physical activity I've described here is safe as long as you do not have a preexisting condition. If you have heart or kidney disease, high blood pressure, diabetes, or arthritis, or if you're currently in treatment for cancer (or have recently completed it), please talk to your doctor before you make major changes in your exercise routine. If you have symptoms, like shortness of breath or irregular heart rate, that make you hesitate before exercising, please check it out with your doctor to allay your concerns.

Finally, remember hydration. For women at midlife, it's not about being thirsty; in fact, Dr. Cohen would tell us that by the time we're consciously aware of thirst, our bodies are already dehydrated. Your joints and muscles will thank you, and you'll perform more comfortably, too!

WE'RE IN THIS TOGETHER

I have the advantage in my practice of being able to talk to lots of women about their approach to incorporating exercise in their lives. Kay, for example, was a longtime walker until one of her knees began causing her pain. She says,

I was inspired to do water aerobics by my mother, who, at 90, leads water aerobics at her retirement center. I go to a class three mornings a week. I have none of the issues of weight-bearing exercise, and the stretch is especially useful to me.

I feel stiff in the morning, because it's morning. But I feel better after class. I walk better, everything feels better. I feel virtuous and better able to focus the whole day. I come out of class with a whole lot of energy, much more than if I'd stayed home and nursed my knee.

Water aerobics is a very social experience, which is part of what keeps me going. I go with a longtime friend; we sing along with the oldies; we tease the instructor. Going with a friend keeps me honest. And if my mother can do it, so can I.

Kay's experience is very different from that of Christine, who plays tennis three times a week. One of those sessions is "cardio tennis"; the other two might be doubles.

Running, chasing the ball—it really doesn't feel like exercise. I think that comes with loving what you do. For some people that might be biking or dancing. For me, it's tennis.

After tennis I feel relaxed, not anxious, like I've run out all my anxiety. I feel happy, like my best self. I feel energized, which is counterintuitive. It restores my inner resources to address other people's needs, like my mother or my daughter. When I can't play tennis, I'm really disappointed and feel deprived. I might go for a run instead, but tennis has really become my game, especially since my kids went to college.

Kathy has always been extremely active. She runs, walks, bikes, and skis, depending on the weather and season; she also lifts weights for bone health. "I run four times a week," she says, "from 3 to 20 miles if I'm training for something big, or around 5 to 10 miles if I'm not."

Kathy is an extreme athlete: She's run two 50-kilometer (31.6-mile) trail runs in the past two years while becoming menopausal. She now credits hormone therapy with better conditioning in the second race, both in training and recovery. The emotional aspects of running are as important as—and interrelated with—the physical benefits.

I feel good when I'm running! I have generally more energy. I run with a good friend, and I run alone. It makes me feel strong and capable, and it grounds me. If I'm alone, it's active meditation time. I contemplate the day and my thoughts and future and relationships.

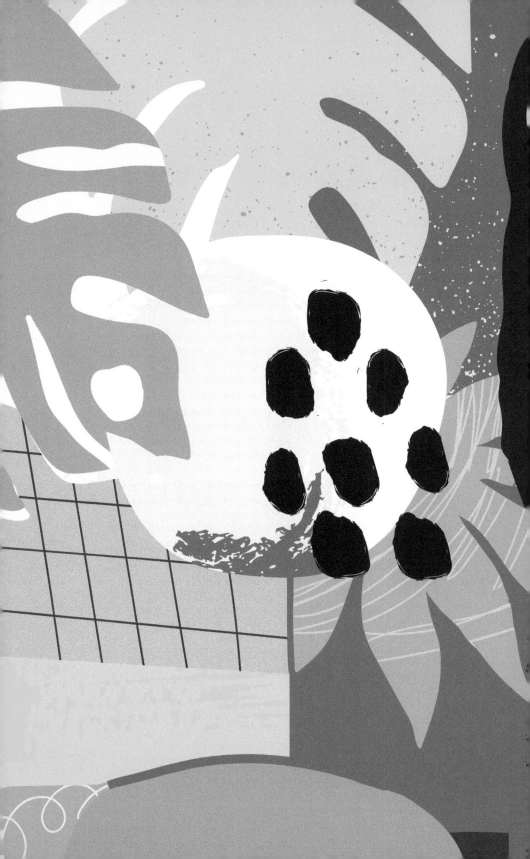

CHAPTER EIGHT

YOUR MENOPAUSE, YOUR FUTURE

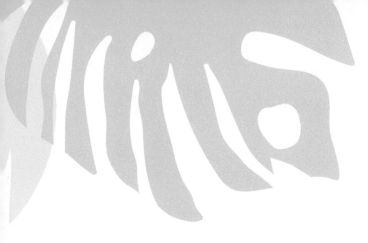

Congratulations on taking the first step toward managing your health and your future! Now that you understand the physical changes that come with menopause, you're prepared to adapt your self-care and advocate for yourself. As women at midlife, we understand our priorities. We've demonstrated how good we are at problem-solving, over and over again. Many of us find midlife to be a time of reinvention, starting new careers or businesses, or diving into new volunteer endeavors.

What these reinventions tell me is that at midlife, we've only just begun.

Keep in mind that while there are general shared realities of menopause, every woman has her own individual experience. You may hardly notice, or you may experience the entire array of symptoms. Perhaps your symptoms started at 38, or perhaps you're just noticing changes at 55. Symptoms may ebb and flow, or be fairly present, for 5 years or for 12. It's all normal, and the most bothersome symptoms are temporary. You'll get through this transition, because women's bodies are amazingly adaptive and highly complex, and you understand how to take care of yours.

If you're just approaching or entering perimenopause, you're in a terrific position to set yourself up for your healthiest menopause transition. By acting now, you can establish the lifestyle and habits that will be a solid foundation for navigating "the change" as it comes. By maintaining or achieving the weight you want to be, you'll minimize metabolic battles in your future. By tuning in to your body now, and even starting your health journal, you'll have a solid context within which to identify and address symptoms as they might occur.

If you're further along in the transition, you can still take the reins! Whatever your starting point, you're equipped with the information and the tactics you need to achieve your best health. All we need to do is make ourselves and our health a priority, worthy of attention, planning, and the time it takes to act on what we know.

We don't need to make this transition alone. I know many of us never heard menopause stories from our mothers. Too much of what we see around us is hot flash jokes of many varieties. I'm seeing the media tide turning, though, with more coverage of women like me and like you, empowered not regardless of, but because of, our age. I'm seeing more articles about the experience and smarts we bring to the table and about the freedom and confidence with which we're living:

- ♥ According to Claire Gill, founder and CEO of the National Menopause Foundation: "Women at midlife are having a moment right now."

♥ In "The New Rules of Middle Age, Written by Women," Candace Bushnell says, "We're not going to do our 50s the way everyone's telling us we're supposed to."

♥ "Changing the Game of Aging" is the subject line of an email from NextAvenue.

♥ In "How I Found My Midlife Mojo," Kimberly Montgomery says, "My world feels like an endless list of possibilities."

Join the conversation. Be sure to talk to your health care provider. When patients speak up, practitioners are motivated to learn more so we can have answers. When you tell us your stories, we understand the impact on real people's lives of topics we may otherwise view through the lenses of research statistics and recommended treatment protocols. I vividly remember a patient describing the effect of her loss of desire on her self-image and her marriage and how it motivated me to press for therapies that could help.

Doctors can advocate for you (and you can advocate for yourself) with pharmaceutical companies, which have begun to make progress in developing therapies for menopause symptoms and conditions but need to do more. They can make clear (and you can, too) the need for more medical research specific to women of all ages and also specifically in the stages of perimenopause and menopause. There needs to be more understanding of the role of the absence of hormones in the last third of our lives and of the risk-and-benefit equations we're all calculating to decide how to manage our health.

This advice doesn't mean you should take responsibility for educating your health care provider. Your OB/GYN may have been terrific during yearly exams or at the births of your children, or you may appreciate how supportive your general practitioner was when diagnosing your appendicitis. That appreciation doesn't mean, however, that they're the right doctor for what you need now.

You deserve knowledgeable menopause care from someone who's well educated in the physical and psychological changes that come with this transition. With a menopause care provider, symptoms are likely to be more readily understood and the role of menopause taken into account. And if you're at all uncomfortable talking to them about symptoms like vaginal dryness or painful sex, that's another sign that it's time to find a health care provider who will be on your side.

If you have a partner, please open communication about menopause. It's important for them to understand how your life, health, and body are changing and how you're reacting to it. If you don't have the conversation, your partner may make assumptions to fill in the gaps. You've committed to each other; there's every reason to believe that your partner will be grateful and relieved to be by your side rather than in the dark.

Every woman's experience is unique, but we can learn from one another, too. One friend may have hot flashes more than you do; she's an ideal teacher of countering tactics. You may have developed some memory cues that work especially well; my guess is that some of your friends would be happy to practice them. Be open with friends about your need to up your exercise routine, and see which of them would like to join you for weekend hikes, nights out dancing, a yoga or tai chi class, or an afternoon bike ride. Share healthy cooking tips, or even develop a shared supper group so you can exchange recipes as well as laughter.

Finally, please engage younger women—your daughters, nieces, colleagues, or neighbors—in understanding menopause as a natural part of life. Eventually, I hope, this part of our human development will be included in our early health education along with puberty and reproduction. The earlier we understand our bodies, the earlier we can begin to manage our health.

You will manage menopause, and you will prevail. We can take charge of our habits and our health. We can find the resources we need to navigate the transition. We can advocate for ourselves and one another! We will care for our amazing, adapting bodies, knowing we are, at midlife, wise, beautiful, and deserving of happiness.

RESOURCES

Fortunately, new products, concepts, and research results are emerging almost daily. As soon as this list goes to print, I'll wish I'd been able to add something. Check the credentials and motivation of resources you find on the Internet; there are plenty of people looking for magic solutions or to profit from this generation of women moving through the menopause transition. The wealth of resources reinforces that although your experience is individual, you are never alone!

Empowered through Menopause

Friend for the Ride is a blog by Barbara Younger that offers "Encouraging Words for the Menopause and Midlife Roller Coaster." **https://friendfortheride.wordpress.com**

The Happiness Project: Or, Why I Spent a Year Trying to Sing in the Morning, Clean My Closets, Fight Right, Read Aristotle, and Generally Have More Fun, by Gretchen Rubin. Another odd choice, perhaps, but I like the encouragement to continue to redesign our homes, habits, and routines, no matter our starting points, to be happy and pursue the lives we intend for ourselves. The author also offers online resources and a periodic newsletter. **https://gretchenrubin.com**

The Moment of Lift: How Empowering Women Changes the World, by Melinda Gates. This book may be an odd choice for a doctor, but I found it inspiring and affirming of our potential as women—at any age, in any place.

The **National Menopause Foundation** is a relatively new organization whose focus is to change the way menopause is perceived in our culture. It offers an online community as well as resources for inspiration and empowerment. **https://nationalmenopausefoundation.org**

Next Avenue offers online community and information resources across the whole spectrum of midlife. Its tagline is "Where Grown-ups Keep Growing," and you can find advice on everything from travel, eldercare, and nutrition to budgeting and career reinvention on the site. **www.nextavenue.org**

General Health

Ask Dr. Barb is my own informational website, where I blog answers to questions I've heard from patients in my practice or that are submitted to the site. A question you have has likely been asked by someone else, and you can join a discussion. **https://askdrbarbdepree.com**

Below Your Belt focuses on pelvic health, including bladder and bowel, vagina and uterus, and muscles and structures. The foundation has developed events, publications, and technology-based tools to encourage women (and girls) to learn about and manage their pelvic health. **https://belowyourbelt.health**

Healthy Women offers health information especially for women, including medically reviewed articles on heart health, diabetes, weight loss, and much more, including addressing symptoms of menopause. **www.healthywomen.org**

Our Bodies, Ourselves: Menopause, by The Boston Women's Health Book Collective. You may remember the original *Our Bodies, Ourselves* as a milestone book for our generation, and this edition focuses specifically on our bodies through the menopause transition.

The North American Menopause Society offers information for women as well as for health care providers. I distribute its *Menopause Guidebook* to patients in my practice; your doctor may, too, or you can order a copy through its website. **menopause.org**

Practical Connections

Estrogen Matters: Why Taking Hormones in Menopause Can Improve Women's Well-Being and Lengthen Their Lives—Without Raising the Risk of Breast Cancer, by Avrum Bluming, MD, and Carol Tavris, PhD. This book is a clear, compelling examination of what we know (and what we don't) about estrogen and our brain, heart, and bone health. I recommend it to nearly every woman who's undecided about hormone therapy.

MiddlesexMD is specifically focused on sexual health, since many of us experience changes. I launched this site when I saw how difficult it was for my patients to get helpful, commonsense answers and products in an environment both discreet and respectful. **https://middlesexmd.com**

National Sleep Foundation offers both educational articles about sleep and practical tips for improving your "sleep hygiene." **www.sleepfoundation.org**

Red Hot Mamas is a multifaceted organization, sponsoring events as well as providing information in their website. Especially of interest may be its links to the ever-changing array of cooling pillows, wicking sleepwear, and absorbent bedding. **https://redhotmamas.org**

Diet

Quench: Beat Fatigue, Drop Weight, and Heal Your Body through the New Science of Optimum Hydration, by Dr. Dana Cohen and Gina Bria. Written by a doctor and cultural anthropologist, *Quench* explains the impact hydration has on things like pain, inflammation, and weight, debunking myths along the way. It also provides a quick-start wellness routine based on new research on hydration. Dr. Cohen makes much of the information available on her foundation's website, as well. **https://hydrationfoundation.org/hydration-guides**

The New Mediterranean Diet Cookbook: A Delicious Alternative for Lifelong Health, by Nancy Harmon Jenkins. You can find lots of cookbooks in this genre by looking for "Mediterranean diet" in the title or subtitle. This one is unpretentious and includes some nutritional information about typical ingredients.

U.S. Health and Human Services offers the classic (updated) dietary guidelines for Americans online as a PDF or as a printed document. If you need a "recipe" to follow to restructure your diet, it could be as simple as this resource. You can also find an electronic copy on Apple iBooks, Barnes & Noble NOOK Books, Google Play Books, and Overdrive. **www.hhs.gov/fitness/eat-healthy /dietary-guidelines-for-americans/index.html**

Exercise

There are too many **yoga apps** for me to review and recommend each one, but I do know the advantages of having a yoga instructor on your smartphone. Search for "best yoga apps" for the current year, and you'll find plenty of reviews to guide you.

AllTrails is a specific app I do recommend. I use it to find walking and bike trails wherever I'm traveling.

Many resources are available to support you as you build your exercise routine. If you're looking for a place to start, you may find this article from **Mayo Clinic** helpful: "Fitness Program: 5 Steps to Get Started." **www.mayoclinic.org/healthy -lifestyle/fitness/in-depth/fitness/art-20048269**

Walk with a Doc is an organization that encourages communities and health care providers to partner for walks that are both healthful and social. See if there's a chapter near you or how to start one at its website. **https://walkwithadoc.org**

U.S. Health and Human Services offers some no-cost online resources that can help develop exercise goals and a plan to reach them. **www.hhs.gov/fitness/index.html**

The **YMCA** offers varied programming in each community, but it's a worthwhile connection to explore. Many offer workout support especially for women, for midlife or older groups, or both; some also include community-building social connection, as well. **www.ymca.net**

Getting Support

American Association of Sexuality Educators, Counselors and Therapists. Sex therapists help couples better understand the role of intimacy and attachment in their relationships and how their verbal and nonverbal communication affects them. This therapy can be especially helpful when, for example, retirement challenges relationship dynamics or physical changes affect intimacy or desire. You can ask your doctor for a referral, or find a nearby therapist through the association's website. **www.aasect.org**

American Board of Professional Psychology, Couple and Family Psychology. Psychological counseling can be helpful in a variety of situations related to midlife changes, including chronic stress, anxiety, depression, or relationship dysfunction. To find a therapist near you, ask your family doctor, or contact the American Board of Professional Psychology at (919) 537-8031. **https://legacy.abpp.org/i4a /pages/index.cfm?pageid=3316**

The American College of Obstetricians and Gynecologists, ACOG's. Don't be put off by the terms of use on this page, which make it look like it's for members only. This directory is free and you can search by state, physician name, or zip code. **www.acog.org/About-ACOG /Find-an-Ob-Gyn**

American Physical Therapy Association. Physical therapists who specialize in vulvovaginal and pelvic therapies can be helpful in treating a number of conditions that may arise through menopause. Your local OB/GYN will know the nearest specialists in your area, or contact the American Physical Therapy Association for a referral to a therapist trained in women's health. **aptaapps.apta.org/APTAPTDirectory /FindAPTDirectory.aspx**

Centers for Disease Control and Prevention. Vaginal tissues are more prone to sexually transmitted infections (STIs) at midlife than at any other time. The Centers for Disease Control and Prevention offers a resource for learning about STIs, protecting yourself and your partner, and getting tested. **https://gettested.cdc.gov**

National Domestic Violence Hotline. Aging can bring changes that frustrate us and our partners. Sometimes that frustration includes anger that can lead to abusive situations. If things have gotten out of hand for you or for someone you know and love, help is always just a click or a phone call away at (800) 799-SAFE [7233]. **www.thehotline.org**

The North American Menopause Society, Find a Menopause Practitioner. Clinicians with the credential of NCMP—NAMS Certified Menopause Practitioner—have demonstrated special competency in the field of menopause. "Find a Practitioner" is a free online referral service you can use to find someone in your area. **menopause.org /for-women/find-a-menopause-practitioner**

REFERENCES

Blumgin, Avrum, and Carol Tavris. *Estrogen Matters: Why Taking Hormones in Menopause Can Improve Women's Well-Being and Lengthen Their Lives—Without Raising the Risk of Breast Cancer*. New York: Little, Brown Spark, 2018.

"Building a Better Body Measurement: Relative Fat Mass." *Cedars-Sinai* (blog). November 17, 2018. https://www.cedars-sinai.org/blog/relative -fat-mass.html.

Chlebowski RT, et al. "Long-term Influence of Estrogen Plus Progestin and Estrogen Alone Use on Breast Cancer Incidence: The Women's Health Initiative Randomized Trials." SABCS 2019; Abstract GS5-00.

Clear, James. *Atomic Habits: An Easy & Proven Way to Build Good Habits & Break Bad Ones*. New York: Avery, 2018.

Cohen, Dana, and Gina Bria. *Quench: Beat Fatigue, Drop Weight, and Heal Your Body through the New Science of Optimum Hydration*. New York: Hachette, 2018.

Davison, Sonia L., Robin J. Bell, Maria Gavrilescu, Karissa Searle, Paul Maruff, Andrea Gogos, Susan L. Rossell, Jenny Adams, Gary F. Egan, and Susan R. Davis. "Testosterone Improves Verbal Learning and Memory in Postmenopausal Women: Results from a Pilot Study." *Maturitas* 70, no. 3 (2011): 307–11. https://doi.org/10.1016/j.maturitas.2011.08.006.

DePree, Barb. "Everything in Life That We Do Is a Balance of Risk versus Benefit." Interview with Carol Tavris and Avrum Bluming. *The Fullness of Midlife*. Podcast audio. January 7, 2019. https://middlesexmd.com/blogs /the-fullness-of-midlife/podcast-risk-versus-benefit.

———. "Learn How to Shrug Your Shoulders." Interview with Joan Vernikos. *The Fullness of Midlife*. Podcast audio. February 25, 2019. https://middlesexmd.com/blogs/the-fullness-of-midlife/podcast -shrug-your-shoulders.

———. "What Subtracts More Than It Adds?" *MiddlesexMD* (blog). April 7, 2014. https://middlesexmd.com/blogs/drbarb/46974787-what -subtracts-more-than-it-adds.

———. *Yes You Can: Dr. Barb's Recipe for Lifelong Intimacy.* Douglas, MI: DePree Women's Wellness, 2014.

The Eating Disorder Institute. "Frequently Asked Questions." Accessed November 12, 2019. https://edinstitute.org/faq.

Fonseca, Angela Maggio Da, Vicente Renato Bagnoli, Marilene Alícia Souza, Raymundo Soares Azevedo, Euro De Barros Couto Júnior, José Maria Soares Júnior, and Edmund Chada Baracat. "Impact of Age and Body Mass on the Intensity of Menopausal Symptoms in 5968 Brazilian Women." *Gynecological Endocrinology* 29, no. 2 (Nov. 2012): 116–18. https://doi.org/10.3109/09513590.2012.730570.

Freeman, Ellen W., Mary D. Sammel, Hui Lin, Clarisa R. Gracia, Shiv Kapoor, and Tahmina Ferdousi. "The Role of Anxiety and Hormonal Changes in Menopausal Hot Flashes." *Menopause* 12, no. 3 (May–June 2005): 258–66. https://doi.org/10.1097/01.gme.0000142440.49698.b7.

Gebbie, Ailsa. Review of "Risks and Benefits of Estrogen Plus Progestin in Healthy Postmenopausal Women: Principal Results from the Women's Health Initiative Randomized Controlled Trial," by Writing Group for the Women's Health Initiative Investigators. *Journal of Family Planning and Reproductive Health Care* 28, no. 4 (January 2002): 221. https://doi.org /10.1783/147118902101196685.

Gordon, Jennifer L., David R. Rubinow, Tory A. Eisenlohr-Moul, Kai Xia, Peter J. Schmidt, and Susan S. Girdler. "Efficacy of Transdermal Estradiol and Micronized Progesterone in the Prevention of Depressive Symptoms in the Menopause Transition: A Randomized Clinical Trial." *JAMA Psychiatry* 75, no. 2 (2018): 149–157. https://doi.org/10.1001 /jamapsychiatry.2017.3998.

Harvard Medical School. "Exercise Can Boost Your Memory and Thinking Skills." *Healthbeat* (blog). Accessed December 4, 2019. https://www.health.harvard.edu/mind-and-mood/exercise-can-boost-your-memory-and-thinking-skills.

——. "Exercise Is an All-Natural Treatment to Fight Depression." *Harvard Health Letter* (blog). Last updated April 30, 2018. https://www.health.harvard.edu/mind-and-mood/exercise-is-an-all-natural-treatment-to-fight-depression.

Hill, Kenneth. "The Demography of Menopause." *Maturitas* 23, no. 2 (March 1996): 113–27. https://doi.org/10.1016/0378-5122(95)00968-x.

Kabat-Zinn, Jon. *Mindfulness for Beginners: Reclaiming the Present Moment—And Your Life*. Boulder, CO: Sounds True, 2012.

Kingsberg, Sheryl A., Susan Wysocki, Leslie Magnus, and Michael L. Krychman. "Vulvar and Vaginal Atrophy in Postmenopausal Women: Findings from the REVIVE (REal Womens VIews of Treatment Options for Menopausal Vaginal ChangEs) Survey." *The Journal of Sexual Medicine* 10, no. 7 (July 2013): 1790–99. https://doi.org/10.1111/jsm.12190.

Müller, Manfred James, Wiebke Braun, Janna Enderle, and Anja Bosy-Westphal. "Beyond BMI: Conceptual Issues Related to Overweight and Obese Patients." *Obesity Facts* 9, no. 3 (2016): 193–205. https://doi.org/10.1159/000445380.

U.S. Department of Health and Human Services. Public Health Service. Centers for Disease Control. National Center for Health Statistics. "Hysterectomies in the United States, 1965–84." Vital and Health Statistics. Series 13, no. 92. DHHS Publication No. (PHS) 88-1753. (Dec. 1987): i–32.

Parish, Sharon J., and Steven R. Hahn. "Hypoactive Sexual Desire Disorder: A Review of Epidemiology, Biopsychology, Diagnosis, and Treatment." *Sexual Medicine Reviews* 4, no. 2 (Feb. 2016): 103–20. https://doi.org/10.1016/j.sxmr.2015.11.009.

Sifferlin, Alexandra. "Why BMI Isn't the Best Measure for Weight (or Health)." *Time*. August 26, 2013. http://healthland.time.com/2013/08/26/why-bmi-isnt-the-best-measure-for-weight-or-health/.

Smith, George Davey, Stephen Frankel, and John Yarnell. "Sex and Death: Are They Related? Findings from the Caerphilly Cohort Study." *BMJ* 315, no. 1641 (December 1997). https://doi.org/10.1136/bmj.315.7123.1641.

Teras, LR, et al. "Sustained Weight Loss and Risk of Breast Cancer in Women ≥50 Years: A Pooled Analysis of Prospective Data." DOI:10.1093/jnci/djz226.

Hanh, Thich Nhat. *Miracle of Mindfulness: An Introduction to the Practice of Meditation*. Translated by Mobi Ho. Boston: Beacon Press, 1987.

Thurston, Rebecca C. "Cognition and the Menopausal Transition." *Menopause* 20, no. 12 (Dec. 2013): 1231–32. https://doi.org/10.1097/gme.0000000000000137.

INDEX

ACKNOWLEDGMENTS

The North American Menopause Society has been an invaluable resource to me, for my own education and certification as a menopause care provider and then as a continuing source of reliable, current, evidence-based information and connections to many smart, like-minded physician colleagues.

I'm grateful to the members of the MiddlesexMD.com team, who support me in advocating for and educating about women's health. Lois Maassen, Marta Hill Gray, and Liz Sitte are especially helpful in keeping me informed, making connections, and occasionally interpreting my medical jargon.

Finally, I will always appreciate my mom's early advocacy for women. Her belief for her own professional worth, regardless of gender, left an indelible impression on me, and I'm honored to carry that banner forward.

ABOUT THE AUTHOR

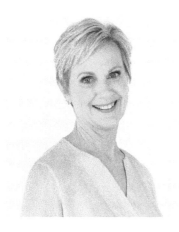

Barb DePree, MD, has been a gynecologist and women's health provider for 30 years and a menopause care specialist for the past 10. She was named the 2013 Certified Menopause Practitioner of the Year by the North American Menopause Society for "exceptional contributions" to menopause care. In particular, the award recognized the outreach, communication, and educational efforts of Dr. DePree as evident in her blog, MiddlesexMD.com. The blog was recognized as one of the "10 Best Menopause Blogs" of 2017 by *Medical News Today*.

Dr. DePree is also the director of women's midlife services at Holland Hospital, Holland, Michigan, where she sees patients regularly. In her practice, she helps women of her own generation—women who are more independent, educated, and assertive about their health than any generation before. She finds that too many of us know less than we wish we did about perimenopause and menopause, which makes the transition more frustrating than it needs to be.

Dr. DePree publishes educational articles regularly on both MiddlesexMD.com and AskDrBarbDePree.com. She lives in West Michigan with her husband and near her three daughters and their families.

CPSIA information can be obtained
at www.ICGtesting.com
Printed in the USA
LVHW070508110220
646443LV00019B/300